TWIST OF FATE

A SWEET SMALL-TOWN ROMANCE

SOUTHERN STORMS
BOOK TWO

LEXIE NICHOLAS

Edited by
KAT NICS

MOUNTAIN WHISPER PUBLISHING

Twist of Fate

By Lexie Nicholas

Edited by Kat Nics
Cover Design by Nickie Cochran

❀ Created with Vellum

CHAPTER ONE

"Stay with me, Cody!" a familiar male voice urged him from far in the distance as he regained consciousness.

His chest was tight and burned as if on fire. Where was he? With each jolt, a sharp pain pierced through his rib cage. The rattling of metal and voices around him calling out medical orders grew louder. He opened his eyes to bright neon lights and water-stained ceiling tiles.

He blinked, then took in his surroundings. Judging by the people walking alongside him, dressed in scrubs and wearing stethoscopes around their necks, and the ceiling tiles zipping past above him, he assumed he was on a stretcher in a hospital. *Not good.* Cody swiped his hand across his face.

The nurse beside him repositioned the nasal cannula under his nose. "Can you breathe all right, Dr. Walker?"

Cody inhaled, then hissed through his clenched teeth as another sharp pain shot through his chest. His heart was racing, and he could hear the blood rushing past his ears with every heartbeat. He blinked twice to focus his vision. "As expected. Thank you."

"Welcome back among the living, Cody," the familiar voice greeted him.

Cody lifted his head, then clenched his jaw as another jolt of pain shot through his chest. "Scott. What…" He lifted his arm and found an IV.

"Relax, buddy. You're at the Emory ER. You've had a heart attack and sailed down the steps at your clinic. From what I hear from the paramedics, you've been in cardiac arrest for a good minute. Thanks to your clinical staff, you're still with us, but I suspect you have a couple of broken ribs and maybe a concussion from the fall. We'll take some X-rays and maybe do a CT to check on all that once we get you settled."

Cody groaned. That explained the excruciating pain in his chest and head every time he moved or tried to take a deep breath. He closed his eyes and focused on being still. He knew he was in excellent hands. Cody had met Scott back in med school in Savannah. Scott, a true adrenaline junkie, specialized in emergency medicine, whereas he found his calling in primary care. Somehow, both their paths led them to Atlanta.

"Which room?" the nurse called out to another behind the nurses' station.

The other nurse turned and checked the board. "Put him in five."

"Hey, Cody, try not to die on me again. I'll check on you once they get you settled in your room," Scott said, then grabbed a chart and disappeared to see another patient.

The ride through the halls of the ER to his assigned

room went much smoother, and he was thankful for that. He hoped he would have a moment of peace to regroup, but he wasn't so lucky. Between the nurses switching out his EKG monitor, lab techs drawing close to a pint of blood, and X-ray taking images of his chest and head, he surrendered to the controlled chaos that surrounded him.

What seemed like hours later, his hands finally stopped shaking once the adrenaline wore off. His nausea also subsided after the nurse injected an antiemetic and pain reliever into his IV and left to tend to her other patients. Cody was finally alone, but he couldn't focus on anything. His brain was restless, yet his body was weak and exhausted. Thinking hurt his head, so he let his mind wander.

As he stared at the wall in front of him and counted nail holes for the tenth time, he noticed the stench of sanitizer and antiseptic cleaner. His clinic smelled a little like that, but not to this extent. At least he knew the place was clean, or at least he hoped so.

Every so often, his nurse rushed into his room to check on his vital signs. "How are you feeling, Dr. Walker?"

"Like I'm ready to get out of here," he said. The bed was uncomfortable, and he was still sore all over, despite the pain medication.

With the noticeable growl of his stomach, he realized he hadn't eaten since he had the two glazed donuts a pharmaceutical rep had brought for breakfast. "Sorry about that, nurse," he apologized. Cody glanced at the clock. It was already noon. No wonder he was starving. "I need to get some lunch."

The nurse checked Cody's chart. "Sorry, Dr. Walker. It says that you can't eat yet."

"Why not? Let me see that chart," he demanded. Cody didn't mean to sound so harsh, but he was irritated, still had a splitting headache, and didn't have the patience to wait. He needed to eat.

Cody tried to lean forward on his elevated bed, reaching his arm toward her and his chart, but the pain in his chest was too intense. He had no choice but to sit back and drop his arm onto the bed again. He glanced at the monitor perched on a rolling stand next to him.

"Dr. Walker, you need to settle down…" the nurse tried to calm him. "Your heart rate…"

"Hey, what's going on?" Scott asked with a frown as he entered the room. "You weren't this grouchy when they brought you in."

"Well, someone's gotta give me some lunch. I'm starving," he grumbled.

Scott shook his head. "No can do. We have to wait for the cardiologist." He glanced over the chart. "Most of your test results came back, and it looks like we have to put in a stent, but we'll let the cardiologist decide."

"A stent? I don't need a stinking stent! I'm too young." Cody could feel blood rush to his head. "What I need is to get out of here and…"

"… and die?" Scott finished for him. His friend's facial expression turned stern. "Because that's what's going to happen to you. You'll die of another heart attack. But I don't have to tell you that, or do I?"

"I'm a physician and can make my own informed decisions."

"And you're also my patient, Cody. Not only do you have blockages in your arteries, but your A1C and glucose tests were also substantially elevated. I hate to tell you this, but you're officially a diabetic. What happened to the athletic hotshot med student who wanted to save the world?"

Cody closed his eyes. Shame coursed through his body. He took a deep breath and winced. His friend was right. He had let himself go over the years. "I bit off more than I could chew, Scott. My patient load has been insane after the staff cuts at our clinic, so the lucky ones that still had a job had to pick up the slack." He shook his head. "I'm putting in eighty hours a week. And forget about exercising. My commute these days is an hour one way with all this city traffic, so by the time I get home, I'm beat. My go-to meals are frozen pizza, deliveries, or I grab a burger on the way home. Then I go to bed and start my day all over again. My life has become a real live Groundhog Day."

"You can't do this to yourself, Cody. This is your body telling you to make some significant changes, or else..." He paused. "It's slowly shutting down. Next time you might not be so lucky." Scott set Cody's chart on the rolling tray. "Dr. Garner should be here soon to talk to you about the stent. My unsolicited advice as your doctor and your friend is to use this downtime and make some tough decisions. I wouldn't want to lose you for something preventable like this," he said and left.

As much as Cody hated to admit it, Scott was right. He often watched his own patients' health, and with that their quality of life, deteriorate from chronic disease before his own eyes. Often, there wasn't anything else he could do if his patients weren't compliant with their treatment. Many of them died a slow death.

Cody closed his eyes. He had to make some major

changes. His life depended on it. Maybe it was time to leave this city life behind. He would give up a lucrative paycheck, but all the money in the world meant nothing if he couldn't enjoy a penny of it—especially not from beyond the pearly gates.

Maybe it was time to pack up his luxury apartment in the suburbs of Atlanta and head back home to Savannah. He'd have to take care of himself and get well first. Only then could he live long enough to save the world again—on a smaller scale this time around.

~

"*H*ere you go, Mrs. Riley," Jenna said, handing one of her loyal customers a box of her weekly order. "Half a dozen double-chocolate cupcakes with cream cheese frosting for Mr. Riley, and the other half a dozen of birthday cake cupcakes with sprinkles for you."

Mrs. Riley smiled and looked at the contents of the box through the clear window of the lid. "They are beautiful, as always, my dear," she said. "Frank will be happy when I bring home his favorite treat."

"I'm sure he will be." Old Doc Porter had made a deal with his patients that they were each allowed one cupcake a week, if they ate right the rest of the time. In Mrs. Riley's case, that meant one cupcake a day. "I will see you next week. Oh, and give Frank my regards."

The old woman nodded at her. "Goodbye, Ms. Jenna. Have a nice day!"

Jenna ran both hands down the front of her ruffled

apron to straighten it. "Whew, it looks like we made it through the morning rush," she said to Beth.

"We sure did. Are our deliveries packed up and ready to go? I'll run them over to Mamaw's Diner before her lunch crowd gets there."

"They are," Jenna said. "Tell Roberta I packed her usual four apple pies and half a dozen of each cupcake variety for her. This should get her through the rest of the day."

Jenna couldn't be any happier with how her shop ran these days. When she opened up her bakery after working years at Mamaw's Diner as a server, it was slow going at first, but as soon as the mayor's wife started raving about how delicious her cupcakes were at a Chamber of Commerce meeting, demand skyrocketed. Add the Hurricane Gerard evacuation crowd out of Tybee Island and Savannah in August, who spread the word about her Hurricane Caramel Swirl cupcakes, and now she was up to her ears in trying to keep up with the demand. But it was worth it to see the excited faces of her customers as they picked their treats and walked out with a colorful cupcake box or two.

"I really appreciate you quitting your waiting job at Mamaw's Diner and coming to work for me instead," Jenna said, "but with all these new customers, we're going to run ourselves ragged. I can't seem to keep up with the baking."

"I was wondering why you're still trying to run everything yourself in the back. You're going to burn yourself out if you keep up this pace," her friend said as she cleaned the glass of the display counter. "We should be able to afford some help, considering how our sales picked up, or no?"

Jenna sighed. "You're right. But what if this increase in sales is only a short-lived? I won't be able to keep another employee if we're having a lull in sales. What if people are getting tired of eating cupcakes?"

"Then we have to get creative and get our customers excited again."

"I don't know, Beth. What if…"

Beth smacked her hand holding the paper towel on the counter and looked her straight in the eyes. "Jenna, you're my best friend, and I say this with love," she began, "but stop it with this worst-case scenario thinking. You know our customers love your baking. We have so many regulars, and they will keep coming back, no matter what. Believe in yourself and your abilities. I do. If we keep going like this, we should worry more about running out of inventory, not customers." Beth winked at her friend. "Sorry, but I had to say that."

Jenna cringed, but she knew her friend was right. She worried too much, and not hiring help soon would hurt them even more. "Thank you for being honest, Beth. I'll think about it."

The bells above the shop door jingled, and a woman in a paramedic uniform entered the bakery. "Hi Jenna. Hi Beth," she greeted them, then stopped to take in the aroma of the freshly baked cupcakes. "I was in the area and couldn't resist the wonderful smell of your goodies, so I had no choice but to stop by and get me a treat."

"That's the whole point, Anna," Jenna said with a wide grin. "So, where have you been? I hadn't seen you in a while."

"I'm sorry; I'm such a terrible friend," Anna sighed. "I've just been so busy with my new job, and we're still revamping mom's Spinning Yarns craft shop."

"And you forgot to mention Jaaaaasoon!" Beth added in a sing-song voice, overemphasizing his name.

The women laughed. "That's Chief Meteorologist Jason Morrison," Jenna teased. "How is he doing, by the way?"

"He still has a small scar left on his forehead, and he has officially passed on the storm chasing baton to one of the younger meteorologists at the TV station. He'll miss it. But after his incident with the hurricane, he realized how dangerous it was—not that he didn't know that before. But his daughter already lost her mom, and this last adventure was too close for comfort."

There was a short, somber pause until Anna broke the awkward silence. "So, Beth, since we're all catching up, how are things with you and Kevin?"

Beth's face brightened with joy. "We're getting married at the courthouse in two weeks." She held up her left hand and showed off her modest engagement ring.

"Congratulations, Beth." Anna paused. "That soon? You just went through a traumatic event."

Beth's smile widened and small crinkles appeared in the corner of her eyes. "When you meet the right one for you, you just know."

"I can't argue with that," Anna said. "Except Jenna had to give me a good talkin' to when Jason and I hit a rough spot."

"Same here," Beth said. "I think we need to return the favor."

Anna and Beth both stared at Jenna.

"Oh, no, you don't!" Jenna said.

"You're the last one of us not in a relationship," Beth said, "and we'll make sure we get you hitched."

"I don't need your help in that department, thank you very much. I can hold my own."

They both frowned at her. "We hate to tell you this, but you're the one who's still single, sweetie."

Beth suddenly froze, looking through the shop door onto the street. Her mouth gaped open. "By golly. He's the one for you."

Anna joined her by the door. "Yep, you're right. That's the one."

Jenna didn't know what they were talking about and moved out from behind the counter to get a better view.

A blue convertible sports car stood in front of Doc Porter's practice across the street. She didn't see many of those in Magnolia Hill. Did some ritzy guy from Savannah visit Doc Porter? Why else would someone drive here in a car like that? Inside the convertible sat a handsome man about her age wearing fancy shades.

"This must be Doc Porter's replacement?" Anna said.

Jenna knew Doc Porter was retiring, but someone who could afford this car wouldn't want to be living in a small town in the sticks like Magnolia Hill. To her it was home, but for city folk like that guy, it would only be a matter of time before he'd climb the walls.

They watched as he got out of his car and disappeared in Doc Porter's practice.

Jenna noticed her heart beat twice as fast.

"That was a nice pair of jeans with that blazer," Anna said.

"Miami Vice, y'all," Beth said with a grin. "Marry

him, and you won't have to work your fingers to the bones anymore."

"Uh, no. Not a chance," Jenna said. "Yes, he looks handsome, but we won't have a thing in common. He's rich, and by the looks of it, he's from the city. I'm the exact opposite. Besides, something doesn't seem right with that picture. I can't put my finger on it, but I have a feeling this doesn't end well. Just wait and see."

CHAPTER TWO

*C*ody grabbed his cup of coffee, flipped the lock of his glass sliding door, and stepped onto his back porch. The morning air was slightly crisp, yet refreshing. He needed a quiet moment because two more obstacles for his backyard ninja playground would arrive today, along with a few guys to help him set up the climbing wall and the frame for his hanging rings.

He sipped on his coffee and scanned his property stretching out into the country. The four acres of land were now his, and he had plenty of room to spread out his equipment. His plans for what he wanted to do with this land were grand. He looked down at his medical alert bracelet. He knew he had to stay healthy so he would be well enough to help his patients. To him, exercise had to be fun or else he wouldn't do it. Working out on a ninja obstacle course was a blast. Maybe some of his patients would be interested in joining in on the fun. But he still hadn't thought out all the logistic and legal aspects of his project—mainly, the liability portion. He'd get to that, eventually.

Cody's cell phone rang inside the house. He stepped back into the kitchen and answered.

"Dr. Walker?" a rough male voice said.

"Yes," Cody replied.

"Mike with the delivery company," the man said. "I just wanted to let you know we will be at your house in about an hour and a half."

"Thank you for the heads-up, sir. I will see you then," Cody said before they ended the call. Good, this would give him time to get in a quick workout and a shower before they'd get his delivery to Magnolia Hill.

Cody looked around the kitchen into his living room area and smiled. The house was perfect for him. It was an older home but had that country charm that he missed living in the city. The cabinets and countertops in the kitchen could use some updating, but he'd take care of that in time. The oak wooden floors were still in great condition, and besides a few tweaks, he was happy. Cody made a mental note to thank his realtor for helping him find this gem. Yes, he was going to have a perfect life on the outskirts of Magnolia Hill, and if he craved city life, Savannah was just a short way down the road from him.

He grabbed a bottle of water from the fridge and set it on the bottom step of his porch. Cody rubbed his hands together, then stretched to warm his muscles. The three obstacles he had set up so far were a modest pull-up bar, a dozen of old car tires lined up flat in pairs on the ground, and a giant tractor tire for flipping. But all that would change with the new arrivals today. He couldn't wait.

Ready to break out in a sweat, he pressed the button on

his watch, then knocked out a few push-ups. He ran to the tires and stepped through them as fast as he could, almost tripping on the lip of one of them. Next he did a few pull-ups, then flipped the giant tire a few times. When he finished his first round, he stopped his watch.

"Not too bad," he said, out of breath. He knew he could do better than that.

He took a few swigs of water and walked a small lap around his obstacles to bring his heart rate down.

His mind wandered to his clinic. Taking over Doc Porter's practice in a sleepy town was just what he had needed. He'd waited a long time for an opportunity to break away from his stressful life that he couldn't refuse. And by the looks of it, he would also be work neighbors with the cute woman with the strawberry-blonde hair at the bakery across the street who always wore that frilly apron. Cody had to smile. Now that his life was less hectic and more balanced, he could see himself taking a chance and going on a date or two again. He'd like to get to know her—if it wasn't for the smell of those fresh cupcakes every day, which was torture for him. He wasn't sure how he was going to handle enduring the tempting aroma that triggered flash-backs of his old life he'd rather forget, but he'd worry about that later.

Back at his porch, Cody checked his watch. "What?" Time must've gotten away from him. That's what he got for daydreaming. Instead of another set of his routine, he knocked out a few burpees, then took a quick shower. With a second cup of coffee in hand, he stepped back onto the porch to envision where he wanted his two new obstacles installed. The last thing he wanted to do was hire a couple of locals to help him lug his stuff around after the crew had left.

The sound of a truck pulling off the road got his attention.

He walked around the side of the house to meet the driver.

"Dr. Walker?" the unshaven man wearing dingy clothes asked as he got out of the truck.

~

A week after his newest ninja equipment had arrived, Cody parked by his clinic as usual, ready to see a full schedule worth of patients. Going to work in Magnolia Hill, however, became more difficult every day he drove onto Main Street. As every morning, the smell of freshly baked cupcakes, pies, and whatever else the woman across the street baked, greeted him. Like one of Pavlov's dogs, he'd almost drool when he got out of his car and the tantalizing aroma of heavenly cakes enveloped him.

He didn't know how much more of the smell he could handle. He'd only taken over the practice full-time two weeks ago, and already he struggled with temptation. Memories of consuming the sweet pastries drug reps had brought to his old clinic tormented him. He couldn't possibly work like this. All he could think of was donuts, and donuts almost put him six feet under a few months ago. He had to remind himself why he was here.

"Focus," he told himself, feeling the resistance of his medical bracelet against his wrist as he shoved his keys in his pocket. "This stuff will kill you."

But his mind had other ideas, and images of those glazed donuts bopped through his mind as if they were floating on a lazy river.

He shook his head to knock those visions out of his mind. If he wanted to live and also to help his diabetic patients improve their health and quality of life, he knew the key was to stay off sugar. He couldn't allow himself to have just a little. To him, those white crystals were the devil—and in his case, like crack cocaine. Even though his cravings had diminished when he started his low-carb diet, convincing his cardiologist of all the new research he had gathered was another task. Most mornings, Cody had a satisfying low-carb breakfast of an omelet with some sausage and veggies, which kept him full for hours and kept his blood sugar levels stable. Over time his blood-work improved. He'd also lost close to forty pounds since the unfortunate incident that brought him to the ER six months ago, with maybe ten or fifteen pounds left to lose. He couldn't focus on what he was missing out on. Instead, he had to remember that he had gotten a second chance at life, and with that the opportunity to help his patients.

Cody entered his practice. "Good morning, Twyla," he said to his receptionist.

"Good morning, Dr. Walker," she said. "Your first patient, Ms. Weaver, is already waiting for you in room one."

"Thank you, Twyla," Cody replied. *Thank God,* he thought, glad to have a distraction from these evil donut visions and cupcake smells.

"Hello, Mrs. Weaver. I'm Dr. Walker. It's a pleasure to meet you," he greeted the woman. "How are you today?" he asked, opening her chart.

"I'm well, thank you for asking, but please, call me Maggie," she said. "And welcome to Magnolia Hill."

"Thank you, Mrs. Maggie…"

"It's Maggie. Just Maggie," she corrected him.

"Well, Maggie, I'm happy to be here," he said as he glanced through her record. "It says here you have type two diabetes. How's that going? Are you testing regularly?"

Maggie shrugged. "Oh, it's not full-blown. Doc Porter said it's just a touch of sugar, and as long as I take my medicine, I'll be fine. He lets me have a treat once a week."

Cody raised his brows at her. "Judging by your numbers, you have more than a *touch* of diabetes." He lifted his eyes from her file and focused on her. "What type of treats are we talking about?"

"Well, I usually get some cupcakes from Jenna's shop across the street. You should try them—they are to die for."

"I'm sure they are…" he mumbled.

"My daughter Anna and granddaughter Ashleigh just moved back into town a couple of months ago, so I get a few more for them. They love them, too. You might have met Anna before; she's a paramedic working for the fire department in town."

He shook his head. "Unfortunately, I haven't had the pleasure of meeting her yet." He counted his blessings that he hadn't needed to call an ambulance to his practice. "But let's talk about your health instead. So, how are those treats working for you? How often do you say you're testing your glucose levels again?"

She blushed. "Maybe once or twice a week when I think of it. They do run a bit high."

"I see." Cody checked her chart again. "Maggie, I also can't help but notice that you've gained a couple more pounds since the last time Doc Porter saw you. I'm not judging, but that's something we need to monitor. Are you taking your medication regularly?"

"I am."

Cody saw complications of diabetes every day at his Atlanta practice and knew from first-hand experience how difficult it was to get a disease like diabetes under control. He'd been there. He smacked his hands on his lap and smiled. "Okay, Maggie. I'm sure you're tired of taking all your medication, and I don't want to increase your dosage. I like to treat my patients conservatively."

She looked at him sideways. "What are you proposing?"

"Okay, here's how it works, and trust me on this. Right now, your body is highly insulin resistant—it can't handle sugar and things that turn into sugar, like starches, very well. That's why your sugar level in your bloodstream stays high. It's just too much. That's why you need medication to bring your glucose levels down. And as you can see, even your medication is having a hard time keeping up. Are you still with me?"

She gave him a slow nod.

"So, your pills are like a Band-Aid. They help with the symptoms, but your body is still overwhelmed with the excess sugar. As a result, when your glucose is high, your body might feel heavy and tired, but at the same time, your mind is restless. A few hours later, your glucose level can take a nose-dive and make you shaky, dizzy, and confused.

I'm sure you've experienced these blood sugar swings before."

"I have," Maggie admitted.

"You can prevent these swings, and I can tell you how. Would you be interested to try?"

She nodded again, but he could tell she had an inkling of what was coming.

"Maggie, by treating the underlying cause of your diabetes, we can help you come off some of your diabetes medications, if not all of them in time. But it requires a bit of work on your part and some trial and error."

Maggie's face brightened. Then it dropped again. "So, what's the catch? Diet and exercise? Don't waste your time. It doesn't work for me."

"No, I want you to try something different." He handed her a sheet. "Don't worry, we'll take it slow. The first thing I want you to do is stop taking in sugar. This means no sweet drinks, like sweet tea or regular soda. Also, no sugar in your coffee and no cupcakes or other sweets."

He saw the disappointment in her eyes. He knew exactly how she was feeling. "I want you to check your blood sugars as outlined on the sheet I gave you. Record your numbers and write down what you had to eat starting today. That way we can see if you're making progress and if we need to lower your medications." He made eye contact with her and waited for a sign of confirmation. "Also, I just wanted to let you know that you also might get a headache after one to two days and might feel rotten for another day or two. This is normal as your body is coming off the sugar and is nothing to be alarmed about. These are withdrawal symptoms. Think of it as akin to quitting smoking or drinking."

"But I love Jenna's cupcakes."

Cody smiled. "It's tough, but if you can do this, we can get you better, and you will have a much easier time getting around. I'm sure Doc Porter had told you that diabetes is a progressive disease, and it slowly gets worse if not managed. I have seen patients lose their feet or eyesight and slip into comas. You can prevent this. Trust me. I became diabetic, and now my blood sugar levels are controlled. I'm living it, and I can help you with this, too. There's a lot of new research that this works."

"No exercise?" She smiled.

"Not unless you want to."

"Okay, Doc. I'll give it a try," she promised.

"That's great, Maggie. We can fix you up. Remember, your body can't handle sugar. Let's keep it out of your diet, and I'll see you next week with your testing results written on that handout, okay?"

She nodded. "Thank you, doctor…I think."

"Don't hesitate to call the front desk and leave a message with my receptionist if you have any concerns before your next appointment." He rested his hands on his thighs. "Unless you have more questions for me, this should do it for your visit today."

She shook her head. "No, doctor."

He stood and ushered her out of the treatment room to the front door. She was a sweet woman, he thought, and he knew her struggles well from his own experience. His heart went out to her. This was something that's fixable.

Cody added a few notes to Maggie's chart, then returned to his office and peeked out of his window. He couldn't believe it when he saw when Maggie heading across the street and straight into the bakery.

His jaw clenched. Didn't she just promise him less than five minutes ago she'd come off sugar? He couldn't blame his patient when he was struggling himself. But he could blame the owner of the shop for poisoning his patients.

CHAPTER THREE

"Only half a dozen of cupcakes today?" Jenna asked, surprised as Maggie usually bought a dozen at a time. "Did the girls not like them?"

Maggie frowned. "They love them, but Dr. Walker put me on a new diet for my diabetes, so I can't have sugar or cupcakes anymore. At least I get to watch Anna and Ashleigh enjoy them. It always makes me smile when I see them happy."

"He won't even let you have one? I'm sorry, Maggie."

The woman shook her head. "Nope. Not a crumb." She handed Jenna the money to pay for the treats.

Jenna could sense Maggie's sadness. She was one of her first customers and always had nothing but praise for her baked goods. Today, her always cheerful eyes didn't have their usual sparkle when she came into the shop. "Here's your change, Maggie. Give Anna and Ashleigh my best," she said, then watched her friend's mom carry out the box of cupcakes to her car across the street.

"So, supposedly our new doc is quite the hit among the

female patients in town," Beth said. "Twyla from his front office told me he's booked up for at least a month."

Jenna turned toward her friend. "I don't think Maggie shares those sentiments, but as long as his patients also buy cupcakes after their appointments, I'm happy."

"As long as he doesn't put them on his special diet too." Beth rearranged a tray of cupcakes on display, then glanced at her friend. "Don't you think he's the least bit cute? I do. But don't tell Kevin I said that."

Jenna smiled. "My lips are sealed. And yes, he's handsome, but he's not the kind of guy I see myself dating."

"Why not?" Beth asked. "He checks all the boxes as far as I can tell. He's very handsome, he's got a convertible sports car, and he's single from what I hear."

Beth had a point, and yes, he was absolutely dashing, but she had no time for someone like the new doc. Going on a date with him would be a waste of her precious time. "I already told you the first time we saw him—he's a rich city doctor, and those guys are shallow and more interested in themselves and their money than someone like me. Believe me, I don't care for all that. I want someone who loves me for who I am, someone who wouldn't mind rubbing my tired feet when I come home exhausted, someone who sits out on the porch with me and enjoys the sunsets before the mosquitos come out. That's the kind of man I want, and trust me, this guy ain't him."

"Is that really what you think? Since when are you that judgy? You haven't even officially met him."

"I'm just not interested," Jenna said, surprised how easily that lie came out of her mouth. "All I know right now is that I can't keep up with my baking, even with your help. On top of that, I'll have to make the cake for the

Miller-Dawson wedding on Saturday." She wiped her forehead with her arm.

"How about the mayor's wife? Clarissa can help. She's a Susie Homemaker."

"The mayor's wife?" Jenna violently shook her head. "No, really, Beth," she grimaced. "You can't be serious."

"Why not?"

"Because I prefer only people I like to work for me. I mean, I appreciate her sending customers our way during my first Chamber meeting after I opened the bakery, but I'll rather scratch my eyes out than have this hoity-toity woman work in my shop."

Beth smiled. "Well, thank you for the indirect compliment," she said, "but right now you need someone with mad baking skills to keep you from burning out, and Clarissa could just do that. She's an excellent baker. Have you tried her peach cobbler yet? It's out of this world." Beth paused, then whispered, "Besides, there's a rumor that the mayor got himself into a bit of a financial bind with buying the Hawthorne mansion last year."

"Ah, I don't know, Beth." She'd hire ten high school kids over the mayor's wife any day. The woman drove her absolutely insane. She was controlling and always had something to say about everything and everyone. "Besides, she already has a full-time job at the Chamber. We need someone who is more flexible."

"She's going through a tough time, and I feel bad for her. That's all," Beth said.

"The answer is no. End of discussion. We'll find someone else," Jenna said. "I don't even know how you could even think of suggesting her." She had to put her foot down on that one. "Just make a sign for baker wanted and post it in the window, please?"

"What about me?" Beth asked. A slight blush colored her cheeks. "I can learn how to bake. I'm not an expert, but I'd like to give it a shot."

"You would?" Jenna asked.

Beth nodded with a wide smile across her face.

"Why didn't you say so before?" Jenna asked.

"You were always so busy…"

Jenna hugged her. "I'd love for you to help me bake; we just have to find time to get you trained. After you come back from making the delivery to Mamaw's, let's hang that sign in the window but change it to say: *Sales Clerk Needed.*"

Beth did a little happy dance, then hugged Jenna again. "Yes! Thank you!"

The front door opened. "I got it," Beth said and rushed to the front of the shop.

Jenna smiled. Why didn't she think of training Beth in the back before? She was a hard worker, and she knew she could count on her. She'd rather teach Beth how to bake from scratch than have to deal with Clarissa any day.

Beth poked her head into the kitchen.

Jenna could tell by her friend's facial expression that something wasn't right. "What's up?"

"Uh, do you have a minute? Someone wants to speak to the bakery owner," Beth said, then pursed her lips.

Jenna put the wooden spoon down on the counter and followed Beth into the store. To her surprise, Mr. Rich Guy was standing behind the counter in his white coat, looking not at all too happy. "Can I help you? My name is Jenna Wilson. I'm the owner."

"Actually, you can. Your store is a major hazard to my patients."

"Excuse me, what?" Jenna couldn't believe her ears.

"Let me get straight to the point. The majority of my patients are diabetic. The smell of the cakes baking in the oven is overpowering them, and they feel compelled to eat. You may not be aware of this, but high doses of sugar can kill them. You need to invest in a better ventilation system to keep the air pollution down."

Jenna coughed, then laughed. "Is this a joke? You can't just waltz into my business after taking over for Doc Porter for a couple of weeks and complain that my baking causes air pollution and the death of your patients. Are you insane? For the record, Doc was fine with his patients indulging in a cupcake every once in a while." She couldn't believe the nerve this guy had. All that money must've gone to his head.

"Simple and processed carbs are very dangerous for my patients, and you are making it very hard for them to keep their blood sugars under control."

Jenna didn't want to argue with someone crazy as Doc Bad Attitude—whatever his name was. "Look, if my baking bothers you, I think you need to aroma-proof your practice or move. Get one of those clean room hoods installed by every door and window in your building and you should be fine. Or move back to where you came from." With a satisfied smile, she turned and walked back into the kitchen, leaving him standing there flabbergasted, in front of the counter "Goodbye, Doc," she called over her shoulder.

"This is not over," he threatened and let himself out of the store.

*J*enna stomped into the kitchen and searched for something to throw. The kitchen towel was closest and least damaging, and she tossed it into the corner with a grunt. It wasn't as satisfying as she had hoped it would be. How dare he come into her store and accuse her of killing his patients? She was right about trusting her instincts all along—he was off the rocker.

Jenna saw Beth poke her head around the doorway. She sighed. "It's safe. You can come in. I promise not to throw anything at you."

"Thanks." Beth nodded toward the front of the shop as she entered the kitchen. "I didn't expect that," she said. "I mean, he just walked in all mad. Trust me, I had my share of difficult customers when I was working at Mamaw's Diner, but this one takes the cake."

Jenna's head was throbbing from the blood rushing to her head. "Don't call him a customer. He didn't spend a penny in my shop." She paced, then lugged an extra bag of flour and sugar from the pantry to the kitchen, but it did nothing to calm her stirred up emotions. "This guy had the gall to insult my business, just like that, without warning, out of the blue. Air pollution? Are you kidding me?"

The corners of Beth's mouth curved into a smile, then she turned away, raising her hand behind her. "I'm sorry, Jenna. It's really not funny and I'm trying not to laugh…"

Jenna shook her head. She loved her friend, and come to think of it, this whole scenario that played out a few moments ago was ridiculous in hindsight. "Yeah, it was kind of funny." Who did this guy think he was? He's new in town, and he walks into another local business that had been there before he showed up in Magnolia Hill, and then claims she was polluting the air.

"Maybe he sniffed too much ether or something in his office."

"That might be a viable cause," Beth agreed, filling the almost empty container on the counter with flour.

Jenna opened the bag of sugar she had set on the counter and refilled the other container. She had made up her mind. She would not think about the crazy doctor anymore and made a note to make her next checkup appointment with a physician in Richmond Hill or Savannah. There was no way she was going to let this arrogant jerk treat her.

Still wound up about the incident, Jenna had to get her mind off what just happened and his threats to shut her down. If he tried, the entire town would have her back. At least she hoped so, because her bakery was all she had to make a living.

Jenna glanced at the front of the shop to see if any customers had wandered in while she was trying to regain her composure. There was nobody there. Good. She put her hands on her waist and smiled. "Beth, are you ready for your first lesson in baking?"

Her eyes opened wide. "Yes!"

Seeing her friend excited like this made her heart swell with joy. Why she didn't take the time earlier to offer her to help was beyond her. "Well, let's start with the basics, then." Jenna grabbed a decorative box from a shelf in the corner. "I don't really go by recipes anymore, but I've written down the final recipe for each cupcake we make, just in case. It's only a matter of pairing the right batter with the right frosting and toppings. So, to start with, we'll make a basic white cupcake batter." She pulled the recipe card for the basic batter out of the box and set it on the counter. "Let's wash our hands first."

Beth did as she was told. "I'm ready."

"Next, we gather all the ingredients," Jenna said, opening the lids for the flour and sugar containers.

"I'll go grab the eggs and butter," Beth said as she hurried to the fridge.

Sure enough, as soon as they got going, the shop door opened. Jenna's heart raced. Did that jerk come back to complain about something else ridiculous? She closed her eyes to prepare herself for the worst-case scenario, then opened them again, ready to fight.

"Hi, Jenna. Are you in the back?" a familiar female voice called out, followed by the beeps and garbled sounds of a radio.

She released her breath with a sigh of relief. "Yes, Anna, come on back."

Anna walked into the kitchen, followed by another paramedic. "Jenna, Beth, this is my new partner, Sandy. She just transferred from an ambulance service in Savannah, so she has more time to study to earn her nursing degree."

"Hello Sandy. It's good to meet you," Jenna said.

"Yes, ma'am. Same here," Sandy said with a smile. "Anna told me all about your wonderful cupcakes, so I had to come by and have a look. I've been studying so much that my brain is craving comfort food." Her gaze wandered to a fresh tray of strawberry double swirl cupcakes. "These look delicious!"

"First one's on me," Jenna said, preparing to put one in a box for her.

"Well, thank you, Jenna. There's no need to box it up." A devilish grin crossed Sandy's face. "I'll have it right now."

Jenna laughed and handed her a pink cupcake with heart sprinkles.

Sandy admired it from all sides, peeled the paper down, then took a tentative bite. She closed her eyes.

Anna, Beth, and Jenna stared at her, waiting for the verdict. "Oh. My. Goodness. Wow! This is delicious. I can tell that we'll be stopping here a lot in the coming months. Thank you so much, and pack me up half a dozen of your bestsellers."

"You're very welcome." Jenna turned to Beth. "Can you get her order ready?"

"Of course. Follow me, Sandy," Beth said and headed with the paramedic into the shop.

Jenna turned her attention to Anna. "By the way, Maggie stopped by earlier."

"Oh, did she?"

"She had an appointment with the new doc," Jenna said. "He's a jerk."

Anna stepped back. "Whoa! What makes you say that?"

Jenna recounted the incident when Mr. Rich Doc burst into her shop, accusing her of air pollution and killing his patients.

At first Anna laughed, but then became serious. "You don't think he's got something up his sleeve, do you?"

There was no way he could be serious about his threats to shut her down. Or was he?

CHAPTER FOUR

*A*fter seeing his last patient for the day, Cody walked to his car. As he opened the driver's side door, he glanced at the bakery across the street. It was a mistake.

Jenna, if he remembered her name correctly, wore her usual frilly apron as she collapsed her chalkboard display sign in front of her shop. She raised her head and glared right at him. With a swift turn she picked up the sign, and, with her chin held high, marched back into her shop.

Dang it, he got caught staring, and he deserved every bit of that icy glare she had shot his way. She had every right to be mad at him. He still cringed about his outburst in the cupcake shop earlier today. Maybe he was too harsh, but for the people of this town, and his own sanity, he would have to stand his ground, even if it upset someone else.

All afternoon, his patients would see him first, then head straight for her shop, only to emerge with boxes full of her sweet, sugary poison, artfully decorated to entice the townsfolk of Magnolia Hill. If he didn't know any better, he would say that she was the town's witch who had enchanted the people with her magical cupcakes. The Magnolia Hill Witch—the name had a nice ring to it.

To be honest, he really wanted to know what all this fuss was about with her cupcakes and try one himself, but he couldn't and wouldn't. He had worked so hard to stabilize his own blood sugars and put his diabetes in remission. One cupcake would send him spiraling down deep into the bowels of sugar hell. To him, that white substance and other processed foods, like bread and pasta, were like crack cocaine. One bite and that monster that was already stirring inside of him would be unleashed. He took a deep breath and got into his car.

He sat for a moment to get himself together. What didn't sit well with him at all was how he had handled the situation this morning. Cody rarely showed his anger, but today he didn't know what had come over him. All his life, he swore not to become like his father—impatient and short-fused. Today he came dangerously close, and the realization made his chest tighten. The pace of his heart beats quickened, and his palms became clammy. His breaths became faster and shallower. No, no, no... he thought.

Cody closed his eyes. "It's not a heart attack," he told himself. "You're not going to die. Calm down." He took a deep breath in, paused, then slowly let it out. Cody took another deep breath and focused on slowing his breathing even more. He continued until his heart rate decreased and his anxiety had subsided.

When he could think clearly again, Cody swallowed hard. He had gotten himself into a fine mess with the bakery owner. Whenever he saw her from across the street, she was always cheerful. The people of this town seemed to like her and always had good things to say about her. He knew he had to apologize to her at some point. It was the decent thing to do.

However, he also found himself in a pickle. A large, juicy one at that. As a physician, he had a duty to be an advocate for his patients' health, not to mention his own. How could he achieve this if he fell into his old addictive behaviors with food that almost cost him his life, and how could he expect his patients to strictly adhere to his advice? If he struggled to stay away from pastries, he knew his patients did the same, especially when they saw the disappointment when he told them they couldn't have sweets anymore. That woman across the street put the entire town at risk with her pastries.

Cody had to come up with a better plan to do something about the shop—for the people of Magnolia Hill. He drove to Mamaw's Diner to do just that.

When he entered the restaurant, a server greeted him.

"Hello, Doc, just you?" she asked with a flirty smile.

He nodded. "Yes, just me."

"My name is Cassie," she said as she walked him to a booth by the window.

The slight sway in her step didn't escape him, but he wasn't here to find a date. He had more important problems on his mind. Besides, he just blew his chance with the woman he really wanted to ask out for dinner. It was the story of his life, and he could only blame himself.

"What can I get you to drink? Sweet tea? A soda?" she asked as he settled in the booth.

"Just water," he said.

She nodded and handed him a menu. "Our special today is the chicken fried chicken with mashed potatoes, white gravy, and green beans. Would you like to try it?"

It figured. Another one of his favorites that would run his blood sugar level through the roof. "I'll just have grilled salmon with green beans and butter on the side. And instead of the potatoes, I'd like a house salad with ranch dressing, also on the side."

She tilted her head, but then nodded. "Yes, sir. I have that out to you shortly."

"Oh, and ma'am?"

"Yes?"

"You don't happen to have some paper and a pen I could borrow?"

She smiled, batted her lashes at him, and handed him one of her pens. "Let me check the office for something to write on."

The door to the diner opened.

Cody glanced up, and to his horror, Jenna entered the diner.

He shrunk into his seat, hoping she didn't notice him, but it was too late. She saw him right away.

Her eyebrows narrowed as she glared at him.

A warm wave of blood rushed to Cody's head.

"Hi Jenna," Cassie greeted her with a notepad in hand. Her expression changed to a frown. "What's the matter?" Cassie hooked her free arm in hers and led her to the breakfast bar.

Cody watched as Jenna talked to Cassie. He couldn't hear what she said, but judging by how her arms flailed, there was no doubt in his mind that it was about this morning. Jenna laughed and threw her hand back up in the air. Then both women stared in his direction.

Yes, he now was certain they were talking about him. He resisted the urge to squirm in his seat. Cody couldn't remember the last time he was in an uncomfortable situation like this. The closest he had come close was when he broke his college girlfriend's heart. She wanted to spend more time with him, but he had to focus on his classes. It was the only hope he had to save his mom from dying of cancer. Back then, he believed that if he studied hard enough, he could research treatment options her oncologist might have overlooked and save her life. In the end, he couldn't save her, and his girlfriend had married a theater major. After his mother's death, he couldn't continue on that path to specialize in oncology. It hurt too much.

One of the cooks set a box on the breakfast bar. "Here you go, Jenna. Just the way you like it."

"Thank, Mack," she said, then turned to Cassie. "I've got to go. See you tomorrow."

"Bye Jenna," Cassie said.

Jenna walked to the door, shot him one last glare, then left.

Cassie walked over to him and dropped the notepad on his table. "Your food should be out soon," she said, her voice monotone and her flirty smile gone.

"Thank you," he said and began brainstorming his options of how to stop her from making his patients sicker. For some strange reason, the cheap plastic pen felt heavier in his hand than it should've.

After he took the last bite of his meal, he sat back and read over his new to-do list:

Step 1: Discourage his patients to indulge in the poison the witch is cooking up across the street. (Use tact)

Step 2: Go to the Chamber of Commerce and file a complaint about the business

Step 3: Contact the Magnolia Hills Times to ask if he can write an editorial column discussing health topics. (Damage sugary treats can cause)

Cody had to do what was right, even if it felt awful and wrong. He only had one major regret. If the owner of the cupcake shop didn't already hate him, she would soon enough, which didn't sit well with him. At all.

∾

"*D*r. Walker, Ms. Weaver, your two o'clock appointment has canceled, and you won't have another patient until three this afternoon," Cody's receptionist announced.

"Thank you, Twyla," he replied. Perfect. He finally had time to implement step two of his plan—to file a complaint about the cupcake shop at the Chamber of Commerce. He'd already advised his patients all morning not to go across the street to buy sweet treats with a fifty-fifty success rate. It was a work in progress. "I'm going to run a quick errand," he said to Twyla as he hung his lab coat on a hook and walked out the front door.

Out of habit, he glanced at the bakery across the street.

Jenna was rearranging the window display, then looked up—right at him.

He cringed, as if he'd gotten caught doing something he wasn't supposed to. But before he could turn away, he was yet again on the receiving end of her angry glare. He deserved it. What disturbed him most, though, was despite their animosity, there was something about her that made him wish things could've gotten off to a better start between them. If it wasn't for her profession, he wouldn't have made such a mess out of the situation, and things might have been better between them. His patients had to come first, though, and that was his reality. He turned away from her and walked down Main Street toward the Chamber of Commerce, grateful for a partly cloudy sky and a comfortable breeze.

A couple of minutes later, Cody arrived at the Chamber building and opened the heavy wooden door. The reception desk was empty, but a waft of overpowering perfume greeted him instead. He followed the aroma down a hallway with offices to the left and right on each side. All were empty, but he heard some commotion in the back and followed the sound.

"Well, ya'll, this is all I have today, and unless there are any new items to discuss, this meeting is adjourned," a shrill female voice said, and several employees with rolling eyes walked past him out of the conference room.

Finally, a slightly rotund woman with big hair appeared and noticed him. "Hello, can I help you?" Recognition dawned on her face. "Oh, you are the new doctor. Doc Walker, right?"

At least he identified the origin of the shrill voice and pungent perfume. "Yes, ma'am. And you are?"

"Clarissa Harrington. I'm the director of the Chamber of Commerce and also the mayor's wife. Welcome to Magnolia Hill."

"Thank you."

"What brings you here today? Are you interested in joining the Chamber of Commerce?"

"Actually, no. I need to file a complaint against a business in Magnolia Hill."

Mrs. Harrington raised an eyebrow and led him to her office. "Please have a seat, Dr. Walker." She sat behind the desk and motioned him to sit on the empty chair opposite from her. "Which business are we talking about?"

In the enclosed room, the smell was even more unbearable, and he had to resist the urge to cough to get rid of the tickle in his throat. *Someone should tell her about her perfume*, he thought. "It's about the Cherry on Top Cupcake Shop."

Surprised, she leaned forward and rested her elbows on the calendar pad in front of her. "May I ask what the complaint is about?"

"The shop sells highly addictive pastries which contribute to the worsening of chronic, progressive health conditions, which can cause death in some of my patients. In addition, the aroma may be too strong for my patients to resist those poisonous products, and they feel compelled to purchase and consume these against doctor's orders."

The woman burst out in laughter. She pulled a tissue from a box and dabbed it at the corners of her eyes. "So, you're saying that Jenna is poisoning the town? You can't be serious!"

Cody didn't understand what was so funny. He had stacks of research to prove that consumption of sugar and starches in already metabolically impaired patients could worsen diabetes and other chronic illnesses, and often result in loss of limbs, vision, or sadly even death. He didn't see the humor. "I am serious. Something needs to change."

Mrs. Harrington composed herself. "So, what do you propose should happen?"

"Ideally, the bakery should close for the safety of the people of Magnolia Hill."

She laughed again. "Doc, I have bad news for you. First of all, the Chamber of Commerce is here to promote businesses. The Better Business Bureau handles complaints. Our closest office is in Jacksonville, Florida, and you'll have to contact them. Besides, I happen to like her cupcakes." She shifted in her seat. "Another thing I want to impart on you, Jenna has a heart of gold and would never hurt a soul. That being said, her bakery has been here before you, so don't you think it's bold to waltz into town and accuse our local business owners of killing your patients?" Her glare pierced right through him.

She had a point, but it still changed nothing about his beliefs. "Thank you for your time and advice, Mrs. Harrington. I will contact the BBB."

"Do what you please, but prepare yourself for battle." She stood, then smiled as if their exchange never happened. "Why, you should come to our next Chamber meeting."

"No, thank you for now. I'm the only physician in town, and I'm sure folks know how to find me." And with that, he left.

He spent his stroll back to the practice by looking up the number for the BBB in Florida on his phone, dialing the number, and explaining his situation.

"I'm sorry, sir," the woman said, "but I'm afraid that your complaint does not qualify for action on our part.

From what I gather, you do not have a marketplace relationship, meaning you did not purchase a product from the business."

"So, what you're saying is that technically, I should buy a cupcake from her and then I can file a complaint?"

"No, Dr. Walker. It means, unless you've been directly affected as a customer, caused by a deficiency of a product or service the business promised to provide, we can't help you."

"So, if I buy a cupcake and have another heart attack…"

"Not exactly," she said.

This wasn't going anywhere, so he ended the call. The only option he had left was to meet with the town's reporter, Miriam Sue Webster, to discuss running a monthly health column in her paper. He might become unpopular, but his patients would thank him one day. And he and his patients would get to live for that day.

That evening, he opened his laptop and typed his first column, his gut twisting as he realized he was likely making things much worse in the name of saving lives.

CHAPTER FIVE

"*T*hank you, for coming in for the interview, Willow. I will let you know if you got the job," Jenna said as she escorted the young woman who'd applied for Beth's sales clerk position to the door. "And be safe tonight. I hear there's some weather coming."

"I will. And thank you for inviting me for the interview," Willow said, then left the bakery, turning back one last time with a smile on her face and her dark blue high ponytail bopping.

"So, what do you think?" Beth asked after the young woman left. "She seemed nice."

Jenna closed her eyes and shook her head from side to side. "To be honest, I don't know." She wasn't too excited about the selection of potential help that inquired so far, but Willow was definitely one of the better candidates. Would her blue hair and black nails scare her customers away? Then there was this issue with the new doctor. What if he makes true on his promise and chases all her customers away? She needed more time to see how things would play out.

"I know it's your shop—and not that I'm complaining, I am very grateful for you teaching me how to bake for the last week—but it's really hard to do both jobs at the same time. We need the help."

Jenna knew her friend was right. Beth caught on fast with helping in the kitchen between customers, and she knew she'd have her fully trained soon, but she had to admit that this couldn't go on much longer. They needed to hire someone to take care of customers during their busiest time in the mornings and the mid-day slump when the people of Magnolia Hill were craving sweet pick-me-uppers for a snack. Jenna sighed. "I hear you. I'll decide by the end of next week. Let's see who else applies. Hang in there, Beth."

"I'll hold you to it," Beth said with a mock stern expression, then greeted the customers that just entered the bakery.

～

*H*ours later, Beth had already gone home, and the store was closed for the day. Jenna stayed late to finish the last-minute wedding cake order for Saturday, but she wasn't complaining. The more she thought about it, though, the more she was ready to call Willow to offer her the job. She sifted the flour into the butter, sugar, and egg mixture and let the mixer do its job. As she watched the beaters swirl the dough in the bowl, her thoughts drifted back to when Dr. Walker waltzed into her shop and threatened to shut down the bakery.

Dread squeezed her chest. What if he was serious? She had worked hard at the diner and saved every penny to afford to open her bakery. Then this guy showed up in town and threatened to end it all. If he succeeded, she'd have to fall back to work for the dragon, Roberta, at Mamaw's Diner, the place Jenna and Beth had worked at together for years and had escaped from. The food was great, and the locals ate there regularly, but Roberta was difficult to work for, to say the least. She shuddered, then paused the mixer.

The music stopped on the radio. "Remember, we have a powerful line of thunderstorms pushing through this evening, some of these storms could become tornadic," a male voice announced.

Jenna walked over to the radio and turned it off, then grabbed a remote and flipped on the small TV in the kitchen just to see the radar. It was time for the news, anyway. Usually, there was nothing exciting happening in Magnolia Hill, and for that, she was glad. But when strong storms were approaching, even later in the season, she paid attention. She got her fill of storm chasing with her friends as a teenager and knew the damage these storms could cause. After several close calls, Jenna now had a healthy respect for dangerous weather.

She poured the batter into the greased and floured cake pans. Once they were in the oven, she set another timer to remind her to check on the cake layers. For now, she would prep a few of the cake decorations ahead of time, and tomorrow she'd assemble everything.

"Hello folks," said the voice on the news. "This is Chief Meteorologist Jason Morrison. I just wanted to remind you that the most western counties of our viewing area are already under a tornado watch until eight o'clock tonight and give you a quick update on the storms heading our way this evening. I wouldn't be surprised if the weather service expands the watch area to include our counties within the hour. We already have some radar-indicated tornado warnings issued to the west of us, so stay weather-aware. This strong line of storms is increasing in strength as it moves into our area and could become dangerous. Our folks out west in Hinesville, Richmond Hill, and the surrounding areas, including Magnolia Hill, will see the weather rapidly degrading around six tonight. For the Savannah area, the storms should begin around six thirty. Keep your TV tuned to this channel for continuous coverage as the first warnings are issued for our viewing area. Again, this line packs quite a punch and rotation has already been observed in several of the cells heading our way, so stay alert and try to get to a safe location if you live in a mobile home or are traveling."

Jenna checked her watch. It was a little after five. She could get the cake out of the oven and let it cool as she cleaned up. With any luck, she could beat the storms home. She was exhausted and really didn't want to get stuck at the bakery longer than she needed to tonight. Besides, a glass of pinot noir and a new book from her favorite romance author were calling her name.

Soon the timer beeped, and the toothpick test confirmed that the cake layers were ready to come out of the oven. She grabbed a kitchen towel, pulled them out of the oven, and after a few minutes turned them onto a cooling rack.

A shrill beep blaring from the TV made her jump. With her hand on her heart, she glanced up and saw an alert banner crawl across the screen. "The National Weather Service has issued a tornado watch until 7 p.m. eastern time tonight for the following counties," a robotic voice said.

Jenna looked at the radar in the bottom corner of the screen and saw that most of the central and eastern counties of the state were in the red shaded area. She didn't think much of it, as these watches were almost routine in the spring and summer, and even sometimes as late as October. But she needed to get a move on if she wanted to avoid getting caught in the mess. Besides, there was no point in starting any baking projects in case Magnolia Hill lost power during the storm.

She cleaned the kitchen and stored the cake layers for tomorrow, then turned off the lights and locked up the bakery. One look at the sky told her she was going to ride right into the storm if she didn't step on it. *Ugh, thanks Jason. The weather got here early*, she thought. For a moment she considered staying in the shop, but relaxing with some wine and a good book was too tempting. She could make it. As she got into her used SUV decorated with her Cherry on Top Cupcake Shop name and logo decals, she glanced across the street. As every night, the new doc was still in his practice when she left. He was more of a workaholic than she was. Maybe she should warn him about the weather. She thought for a second. "Nah." He could fend for himself. He probably knew about the tornado watch already, and by the looks of it, he wasn't going home anytime soon, anyway.

The air pressure had changed, and her ears were popping, which wasn't a good sign. Everything around her took on a greenish hue, and for a moment, everything went silent. Even the birds stopped chirping. She put her car into gear and drove off. If she hurried, she could make it. The voice in her head was begging her to turn around and warn Doc, but she ignored it.

It turned dark within minutes, and the lightning lit up the sky in front of her. The thunder became louder with every mile she traveled west. She could now hear the distant wail of the town's tornado sirens behind her. "Crap!" Jenna was now on the county road which took her through a wooded area, so she couldn't see the weather in front of her. She gassed it. She was almost home and prayed that she could make it inside her house and to safety in time.

"Only half a mile," she told herself. Lightning flashed ahead of her, followed by an almost instant crack of thunder.

Jenna's pulse quickened. She glanced at her speedometer and realized she was already doing 70 mph on a 55 mph stretch of the country road. Jenna didn't care. She had to get home. Now.

Finally, she pulled into her driveway and drove her SUV under the carport. She pushed her car door open, got out, and slammed it shut.

Loud cracking sounds came from the woods, but she couldn't pinpoint them.

Jenna held her hand on her chest. Her heart was beating so hard that she could feel it in her throat. The pine trees around her were waving and bending in the wind. Then, to her horror, she heard it—the classic sound of a train. The pines just a few yards ahead of her snapped in half like twigs. She braced herself. "Oh my God, oh my God!" was all she could utter when she saw the twister cross the road to the right of her property. "Oh my God! No!"

A powerful gust ripped the sturdy metal carport and slammed her against the wall of her house, where she collapsed onto the cement patio.

And as soon as the twister had come, it had left.

Jenna opened her eyes and stared at the grill of her car only a foot from her face.

She tried to move. The back of her head hurt. *Pain is good*, she thought. At least she was alive. She tried to move her arm, but as soon as she did, a sharp pain coursed through her left shoulder.

She had to get unstuck. Jenna tried to wriggle her way out of the small gap that was left between the wall and her car, but it was too painful to move. She was pinned.

Then she remembered she had tucked her phone into her back pocket. Praying that it was still there, she reached for it with her good arm, but of course it was in her other pocket.

She shifted her butt toward the right. If she could expose the microphone, she might be able to use voice commands to call for help. "Call 911!" she yelled.

Nothing happened.

She tried again with lowering the pitch of her voice and annunciating her words better.

Nothing.

After her tenth attempt, she gave up. How could she have been this careless? She knew tornadoes were nothing to take lightly, yet she was too much in a hurry to get home, and now she found herself pinned outside her own home, wounded and stuck. Who would come find her?

Then she realized that not a soul would have a reason to come look for her.

A large raindrop landed on her nose as to add insult to injury. When the rain turned into small hail, she raised her head one more time.

"Help!" she called out, then sobbed.

~

*C*ody heard sirens go off, looked out of the window and got a glimpse of a twister in the distance until it disappeared from his view behind the buildings across the street from him. There it was—the classic train sound. The only thing he wished he had right now was a basement or storm shelter. He ran to the bathroom closest to the center of his practice, hunkered down, and braced for the worst. The twister didn't move his direction, but there was no guarantee that the storm wouldn't spawn another one right on top of him. Better safe than sorry, he thought, especially when the wailing of the sirens and the howling of the wind continued outside his practice.

Soon, he realized that the sound moved away from him, followed by the clicking of hail hitting the metal roof of his building. Well, there went his car. At least he had the foresight to put the top on when he heard his patients talk about the storm heading this way. Hopefully, he still had a house to go back to.

The sirens stopped. Either the twister took them out, or the danger was over. He checked the radar on his local weather app. Relieved, he saw that the worst weather had passed and was now east of Magnolia Hill. All that followed was rain.

He waited for the hail to stop, grabbed some extra medical supplies just in case, and headed out.

Cody locked his practice and examined his surroundings. His car had a few minor battle scars and a small crack in his windshield, but that he could get fixed. He looked across the street; Jenna's SUV was already gone, and the bakery was dark. The few people that were still downtown looked somewhat shaken up, but other than some wind and hail damage, everything seemed to be okay.

"I saw the twister from my office upstairs," Mr. Boden, the realtor, said with his arm stretched to the wooded area west of town. "It was about a mile or two away, heading northeast of us," he said.

"That's close to my house," Cody said. "I'll drive out that way, in case someone needs medical attention." He got into his car and headed west out of town, keeping his eyes open for anyone injured. There was no telling how long it would take an ambulance to get out here.

The closer he got to the woods and his house, the more debris he had to negotiate on the road. There were tree branches, twisted metal roofs, and lawn chairs scattered all over the place. His primary concern was downed power lines. The last thing he needed now was to be electrocuted.

Cody could see that something large and white was blocking the road about half a mile ahead of him. As he got closer, he realized it was an upside-down carport that landed on the road. Just beyond the carport, trees lay snapped in half along what he assumed was the path of the tornado.

Once he reached the carport blocking the road, he pulled over, hoping the twister didn't injure the person who the carport belonged to. He saw a narrow driveway between two draining ditches. It led to a house set toward the back of the land close to the wood line. A fallen tree blocked the entrance to the property. He grabbed his medical bag and climbed over the tree trunk.

As he got closer, he realized the SUV that stood on a cement pad resembled the car that was always parked across the street from his practice—the one Jenna was driving.

A lump formed in his stomach. How did he miss her SUV parked at this house, even after driving by it every day for the last few weeks? "Please don't let her be hurt," he whispered.

Cody picked up his speed and jogged the rest of the way to her car. "Hello? Anybody here? Jenna? Jenna Wilson?"

He heard a small whimper. "I'm here."

Adrenalin rushed through his body. Cody followed the sound of her voice. When he arrived beside her vehicle, he got a glimpse of her wet, strawberry-blonde hair and the ruffles of her apron plastered against her shoulder. It was Jenna, pinned between the wall and her car. Her eyes revealed a mixture of relief and distaste.

"It's me, Cody—uh, Dr. Walker across from your shop," he said.

"Uh," she moaned and rolled her eyes at him.

He didn't like the sound of it. "Tell me where you're hurting!"

"My shoulder and my head," she said.

Cody did a quick check of her pulse and vital signs as best as he could, then checked her shoulder. "It looks like it's dislocated. Where does your head hurt?"

She motioned with her good arm to the back of her head.

He gently ran his hand along the area she pointed at. "You're not bleeding, but you got a fairly large goose-egg. Did you lose consciousness?"

"I don't think so," she said.

"Let me call an ambulance and some help to get you out from under your car," Cody said and dialed 911 on his cell phone.

A few moments later, he crouched down beside her again. "Help is on the way," Cody said, "but it might take them a minute to get here." Cody looked around. "Do you have the keys your car?"

"Weddin' cake,"

What? Did she just say wedding cake? He smiled. "Don't you think it's a bit too soon to think about that right now, I mean, I like you…"

She rolled her eyes. "No, not ours, dork, and the feeling is not mutual."

Cody couldn't be any happier. She got her spunk back. She'd be okay.

"Keys?" he asked again.

"I don't know," she said. "I had them in my hand when the tornado came."

Cody searched the area under and around her car but came up empty.

A siren sounded in the distance.

"Sounds like help arrived faster than expected," he said, watching as a Sheriff's vehicle pulled up behind his car.

The sheriff jumped out of his car and hopped over the tree trunk blocking her driveway. "Jenna!"

"She's right her, Sheriff," Cody said to the clearly distraught man. "She'll be fine. We just need to move her car back a couple of feet."

"Thanks Doc," he said, kneeling next to Jenna. "What happened? Why were you out in this weather?"

"I thought I could make it home," she said.

Sheriff Oakley shook his head. "You should know better than to outrun a twister," he scolded her, then nodded at Cody. "Let's move this car. Jenna, where are your keys?"

"I don't know," she answered.

"Doc, can you see if the car is unlocked?"

Cody rushed to the driver's side door and pulled the handle. To his relief, the door opened, and he got in. "I'm putting it in neutral," he said. "Let me know when you're ready for me to come off the brakes."

The sheriff stood by the hood and nodded. "I'm ready."

Cody eased off the brake pedal while the sheriff pushed the car back about five feet.

The sheriff held up a fist to signal they were good.

Cody put the car in park again and got out of the driver's seat, then joined Sheriff Oakley next to Jenna, assessing the rest of her body to make sure he didn't miss any other injuries.

"Listen, Jenna," Cody said. "You have to keep your neck still until the medics arrive. We have to make sure you don't have a spinal injury."

"What were you thinking, Jenna?" Sheriff Oakley asked, pacing back and forth on the patio. "You always have such good judgement. This is so unlike you to drive into a tornado, especially after we almost got picked up by one as dumb teenagers storm chasing with our friends."

Cody put his hand on Sheriff Oakley's shoulder. "I don't think this is helping right now."

Jenna smiled. "We got lucky then, Sean. And technically, I made it home."

"Just not inside," the sheriff finished for her. "By the way, that half-rotten pine tree in your backyard landed on your house."

Jenna closed her eyes. "Great."

Cody heard the ambulance and a couple of firetrucks approach. "Do you hear that, Jenna? Help is almost here."

She nodded.

"I need a c-collar and a backboard," Cody shouted out to the medics who climbed out of the ambulance.

"Where's Jenna?" one paramedic asked as Cody met them halfway.

"In front of that SUV, against the wall," he said. "Thank you for coming this quickly. I'm Dr. Cody Walker. I took over Doc Porter's practice in town."

"Oh, we know, Doc. I'm Anna Weaver."

Yep, small town, he thought. "Ah, Maggie Weaver's paramedic daughter, I assume. Nice to meet you."

"I'm here for my friend Jenna and to do my job," Anna said, "not to exchange niceties."

A friend of Jenna's. "Of course," Cody said.

As the paramedics stabilized Jenna's neck, lifted her onto the backboard, then onto the stretcher, Sheriff Oakley turned away as to try to keep his composure.

Cody knew what it was like in a small town where everybody knew everyone. They looked about the same age. No doubt, they grew up together.

Jenna groaned. "How am I going to get the wedding cake done for Saturday? What about my business?"

"We'll figure something out," Anna said as she strapped her on the stretcher.

A tear rolled down the side of Jenna's face. "I can't disappoint them."

"Not now," Cody said. "Your health comes first, okay?"

Cody grabbed a gauze pad and wiped that tear away for her. As he did, their eyes locked.

The other paramedic next to him coughed and smiled. "Uh, Doc, we're ready to take her to the ER."

"Right," he said. He smiled at Jenna, then walked alongside her stretcher to the ambulance.

"Wait, I found her keys," Sheriff Oakley called after them and rushed to catch up. "Argh!" He clenched his jaw in pain.

"What happened," Cody asked.

Sheriff Oakley looked down and pointed at his left foot he had lifted from the ground.

Cody saw a large nail protruding from the sole of his shoe and winced. "Ouch!" He rushed to his side, took the keys and shoved them in his pocket, then stepped to the sheriff's side to support him. "Let's get you to one of those vehicles and get this looked at. We might have to get you to my practice to get the wound cleaned up properly. The good news is that it's your left foot."

As Sheriff Oakley made arrangements to have someone follow them with his vehicle to Cody's practice, Cody watched as the paramedics loaded Jenna into the ambulance, shut both doors, and drove off.

"Do you think she'll be all right, Doc?" Sheriff Oakley asked.

Cody nodded.

CHAPTER SIX

*B*ack at his practice, Cody cleaned the sheriff's puncture wound and wrapped his foot with a gauze bandage. "I checked your record, and it's been twelve years since your last tetanus shot, Sheriff Oakley. Since you're already here, we'll get that taken care of."

He cringed. "Can't it wait, Doc? I'm not a fan of shots."

Cody suppressed a smile. "Sheriff, with this rusty nail going through your foot, you don't want to risk tetanus. Trust me on that."

"You can call me Sean. Can't we postpone it until next week?" he asked.

"Nope. Now roll up your sleeve!" Cody filled a small syringe with the vaccine and cleaned a spot on Sean's upper arm with an alcohol wipe. "Small stick."

Sean pinched his eyes shut and hissed through his teeth in anticipation.

Cody laughed. "I didn't even start yet."

Sean cautiously opened an eye, looked at his arm, and let out a sigh of relief.

As the sheriff looked away, Cody took the opportunity, and with a swift stab and a squirt, injected the vaccine. After many years of coaxing kids to give them their shots, he learned it was all about distraction and timing. He also had learned that adult punches hurt more than those of toddlers.

"Ah!" Sean screamed.

"All done," Cody said, suppressing a grin, and stuck a Band-Aid on his arm. "Come see me in about a week so I can check on your wound. I just want to make sure it doesn't get infected."

"Thanks, Doc," Sean said as he lowered his good foot onto the floor. "And let's keep my fear of needles between us."

"Patient-doctor privilege. My lips are sealed." He followed up his statement with a zipping motion across his mouth. "And since we're now on a first name basis, call me Cody."

Sean rolled his sock over the bandaged foot and attempted to fit it in his shoe.

"Wait." Cody left the room and returned a few moments later with a medical shoe in his hand. "Wear this for a few days until your wound has healed some."

Sean took the shoe and fastened the Velcro straps and got up. "Thanks, Doc—sorry, Cody." On the way out the door, he turned to him with a sly smile. "So, what was that look between you and Jenna before the ambulance took her to the ER?"

"What do you mean?" Cody asked.

"Oh, just wondering. Thanks for fixing my foot," Sean said, grabbing his left shoe. "I'll see you in a week," he said, then left.

Cody walked out of the treatment room into his office and sat on his chair. Leaning back, he let the evening's events replay in his mind. He knew exactly which look Sean was referring to before he left—the one when he wiped the tear off Jenna's face before the paramedics took her to the ambulance. As their gazes had met, something happened to him at that moment, and he wasn't sure what to make of it. After all, she was still the reason many of his patients had such a tough time keeping their diabetes under control.

Even though they were not on the best of terms, he still worried about Jenna. Maybe he should check on her. Would it be wise? Maybe not, but he didn't like things hanging up in the air when all he had to do was make a call. The longer he sat and pontificated, the stronger the urge to check on Jenna became.

He scanned the cork board by his desk for the number of the ER the medics took her to. When he found it, he lifted the receiver off his desk phone, then hesitated. He had nothing else to do, so why not drive out there? Under normal circumstances, he would've stuck to the phone call, but he wanted to check on her personally. That last moment he saw her unsettled him. Maybe there was something there. Maybe there was hope that they could find some common ground one day. They just had to get to know each other better. But that was probably a bad idea, too.

Cody grabbed his keys off the desk and shoved them in

his pocket, noticing that another set of keys already filled that space. "Jenna's keys." He smiled. Now that he had a legitimate reason to visit her, he locked up the practice, and headed to Savannah to check on Jenna—no, to return her keys.

As he entered through the automatic double-doors of the emergency room, the familiar smell of medicine, sanitizer, and a light hint of vomit assaulted his nostrils. The bright neon lights in the ceiling brought back the memory of his unfortunate episode six months ago. Technically, his cardiac arrest could be considered a brief trip into the afterlife, but downplaying it sat better with him. Cody flipped the tag of his medical alert bracelet over a few times. Touching the smooth metal gave him peace and also reminded him he had made it through. He approached the reception desk.

"Can I help you?" the receptionist asked.

"Yes, I'm Dr. Walker. I'm looking for Ms. Jenna Wilson. Is she still here?" He didn't like to play the doctor card, but it would get him where he needed to go—at least he hoped so.

The woman clicked away on her keyboard, then looked up at him again. "She's in room six."

He looked around, not sure which way to go. "Can you point me in the right direction? I don't come here a lot."

The woman paused, then stood. "Follow me, Dr. Walker." She took him halfway down a long hallway. "Take the next hall to the left, then her room is the third one on the right."

"Thank you, ma'am," he said and hurried around the corner in case the woman would start asking questions.

The door of room six was open, so he poked his head

in, hoping she wouldn't throw anything at him. If she did, he well deserved it.

~

*W*ith her arm immobilized in a sling-like contraption, Jenna sat propped up on her bed, waiting for the doctor to return with the X-ray results. Despite the pain medication the nurse gave her through the IV port in her other arm, a dull throbbing pain still pulsed through her shoulder, but her headache finally began to subside.

A million thoughts rushed through her mind. Who was going to finish the cake for Saturday's wedding? What about her shop? Beth? She couldn't close the shop and let her best friend down, leaving her without pay until she'd be well enough to bake again. The only way she knew to calm her racing thoughts was to call Beth.

The nurse had moved her purse to the rolling tray beside her bed but pushed it aside when she got her IV started. Just the thought of stretching to reach for it, though, was daunting. She had tried earlier, but the pain in her shoulder told her it wasn't a good idea.

Jenna looked for a call button, but of course, it was out of reach, too. Maybe she'd see her nurse walk by her door and call out for her then. In the meantime, she'd just have to be patient.

While waiting for her opportunity to get her phone back, she made a mental list of priorities.

1) The shop: Hire help ASAP - Willow?

2) The car port and tree on the house: Call insurance tomorrow.

3) Make thank you calls to Anna, Sean, and maybe Doc Walker—or not.

That last item on her list remained to be seen. She still wasn't sure if she could forgive him that easily after that outburst. Besides, it was his job to save people. Wasn't that part of his doctor oath?

Out of her peripheral vision, she noticed someone standing inside her door frame. In hopes it was her doctor putting her out of her misery and letting her go home soon, Jenna glanced up. Her facial expression fell. *Speaking of the dev*il: also known as Doc Walker. "Oh, it's you," she uttered.

"Hi. May I come in?" he asked.

"Sure." She wasn't in the mood to put up a fight. "Why are you here?"

He sat down on the stool by the sink. "I just wanted to check on you and see if you needed anything." He held up her keys and dangled them on his fingers. "And I also wanted to bring you these," he said, setting the keys next to her purse.

"Oh," she said. "Well, thank you for bringing them to me." Jenna thought for a moment. "Can you push that tray with my purse closer to where I can reach it? I need to call Beth to make arrangements for the bakery."

"Of course." Doc Walker stood and rolled the tray to the side of her bed and handed Jenna her purse. "You look like you're still in pain, and by the looks of it, they didn't pop your shoulder back in place yet."

"We are still waiting on the X-ray results. And," she hesitated, "thank you for helping me earlier."

"You're welcome. That's what I do. Good news is that once they set your shoulder, you should feel much better."

He shifted uncomfortably. "Look, I'm sorry about how I burst into your shop the other day…"

Her doctor stepped into the room. "Ms. Wilson, I have your X-ray report back. Oh, hello, sir. I'm Dr. McSmith," he said, reaching out his hand.

Doc Walker reciprocated. "Dr. Cody Walker. I recently took over Doc Porter's practice in Magnolia Hill."

"Ah, nice to meet you, doctor. I assume you're Ms. Wilson's physician?"

"Absolutely not!" Jenna said. "I will see Dr. Garner in Richmond Hill." In an instant, she regretted the words that shot out of her mouth and the resulting awkward silence. "Dr. Walker helped me after the tornado ripped my carport off the property."

"I live a mile past her house and found her nose-t—nose with her car. I just came to bring Ms. Wilson her keys and see how she was doing or if she needed anything."

Dr. McSmith looked at him, confused, then turned to Jenna. "Good news, Ms. Wilson. The X-rays show that you didn't break any bones, and yours is a simple dislocation. With a treatment called reduction, we can gently rotate your arm back into place. I will give you something for the pain, reset your shoulder, and then we will take another X-ray to confirm everything is good to go before we release you."

Jenna could feel panic spread throughout her chest. The fear of the impending pain made her hands shake and numb. Her breathing quickened. She glanced up at Doc Walker.

"Don't worry, Jenna. With the pain medication, you'll just feel some pulling and tugging."

"If you say so," she replied, but wasn't sure if she could trust him.

Dr. McSmith injected her painkiller through her IV port. "Let's give this a few minutes to work, and I'll be back to set your shoulder."

Jenna still couldn't relax. "Doctor Walker?" she asked.

"You can call me Cody."

"Cody? Will it hurt? I mean, you're a doctor, and you've done this before," she said, her voice shaking. The ambulance ride was painful enough, and the thought of moving her arm made her cringe.

He moved closer to her bed. "It won't. I promise."

Jenna glanced down at her phone. "I have to call my friend before I get sleepy. Do you mind?"

"Not at all," he said with a reassuring smile. "I'll step outside so you can have some privacy."

"Thank you," she said and selected Beth's name from her recently called list on her phone.

"Oh my gosh, Jenna! Anna told me you got caught up in the tornado. Are you okay?" Beth asked.

"I will be," Jenna said. "I have a dislocated shoulder, a nice goose egg on the back of my head, and a few scrapes, but otherwise I'm okay."

Beth let out a sigh of relief. "I was worried sick about you."

"Hey, listen, I don't know how much time I have to talk, but can you do me a huge favor?"

"Anything, you need," Beth said.

"As much as I don't want to do this, but can you call Clarissa and ask her if she could help finish the wedding cake? Everything is ready, she just has to assemble it and make it look pretty. Also, can you ask her if she could help in the mornings to decorate some cupcakes while I can't move my arm?" All she could think of was how much she didn't want Clarissa under foot. But Beth was right; the mayor's wife, as annoying as she was, could bake up a storm. Every year she won several pie contests during the town's fall festival, and this year hadn't been an exception. *Oh, Beth, why did you have to suggest her?* she thought, making a mental note to strangle her tomorrow, or thank her. Maybe she should thank her first, then strangle her when Mrs. Mayor became a pain in the neck.

"Don't worry, Jenna, I'll call her. We'll work something out," Beth said.

"One more thing," Jenna said with a smile. "You'll be proud of me."

"Oh?"

"Can you call Willow and offer her the sales job? We can do all the employment paperwork on Monday."

Beth squeaked on the other end. "Finally! It took an act of God for you to hire some help."

"I'm sorry it took me so long to decide," Jenna said. A sense of guilt swirled around in her stomach area, or maybe it was the painkiller making her queasy. But she had to admit, Beth had to pull double duty for way too long. She should've set her perfectionism aside long ago and not been so picky about hiring the perfect staff at the cost of burning themselves out.

"The bakery is your baby. You've worked so hard for it. I get it, Jenna," Beth said. "Don't worry about the shop. Oh, and call me if you need a ride home. I'll come out and get you."

As soon as Jenna ended the call, Dr. McSmith returned

with Doc Walker in tow. "How are you feeling, Ms. Wilson?"

"Scared," she admitted.

"Don't be," Dr. McSmith said. "We'll get you feeling much better in a few minutes. Let's remove the sling, first."

Jenna reached out to Cody with her good arm.

He took her hand into his. "Just focus on me, okay?"

CHAPTER SEVEN

"You're all set, Ms. Wilson," Dr. McSmith said an hour later. "Your X-rays are back, and your shoulder looks great. Your nurse will take out your IV and go over your discharge instructions with you. I will send your prescriptions over to your pharmacy."

"How long do you think will it be before I can use my arm again? I run a cupcake bakery," Jenna asked.

"You'll need to rest and keep your arm still for at least a few days. Your doctor might let you return to light duty in two weeks. Full recovery might take eight to twelve weeks."

Jenna let out a sigh. "Two weeks?" She let the words sink in. "My bakery!" How was she going to keep her business going? At least she'd have to pay her rent and Beth's wages. Add Willow's and Clarissa's wages, too. Her head spun.

"I'm sorry, but you have to let your shoulder heal. With

rest and some physical therapy, you should recover well, though." Dr. McSmith left the room.

Jenna turned to Cody. "What time is it?"

"Almost midnight."

She groaned. "It's too late to call Beth to take me home."

"No worries," Cody said. "I'll give you a ride. Your house is on my way, anyway."

"Thank you," Jenna said. "I'll text Beth, so she won't worry." Jenna was glad that he came and stayed with her. There was something about him that made her feel at ease. She shouldn't let her guard down, but what's the worst that could happen? He was only giving her a ride home.

After she set her phone aside, she noticed that her mouth felt dry. "Can you get me something to drink? I'm suddenly so thirsty."

He handed her the plastic cup with water the nurse brought in earlier. "Here you go." He sat in the chair next to her bed.

After almost finishing the half cup of water, Jenna smiled. "Thank you for doing all this for me. You really didn't have to." Out of all people, she didn't expect him to check on her. She thought he would be some sort of non-caring, big city, rich guy, especially after he was going nuts on her that first time they met. Instead, his kindness threw her for a loop.

He reached for her hand, squeezed it, and let go, as if he realized he'd made a mistake. "My pleasure."

Maybe it was for the better. Her focus now was on making do for the next two weeks. Jenna wasn't looking forward to dealing with all the fallout from this storm. "Has Sean mentioned something about my house yet?"

He shook his head. "I haven't heard from him. Let's get you discharged first, and then we can check on it when I drop you off and get you settled."

A woman with a clipboard entered the room. "Hello. I'm Sonya from billing. I just need a signature from you before we send you on your way. How are you feeling, Ms. Wilson?"

"Much better, as far as I can tell."

"That's good to hear," Sonya said with a smile and handed her the clipboard. "I just need you to sign here on the bottom. Then your nurse will be back with your discharge instructions. She said your companion can pick up your medication from the inpatient pharmacy to hold you over until the morning."

He grinned at her.

What she wanted to tell Sonya was that he was only her ride, but she gave up and let it go instead. With one hand, she dug in her purse for her wallet, pulled out her driver's license, and handed it to Cody.

When he came back with her medicine twenty minutes later, she was already dressed and sitting in a wheelchair.

"Dr. Walker, I have her discharge instructions in this envelope," the nurse said, handing him the papers. "Ready?" she asked after she rattled off the highlights of her aftercare.

Jenna nodded. She was glad to get out of the hospital, but her legs were still wobbly when Cody helped her into his car. After that evening's ordeal, Jenna couldn't be any happier to get home and get some sleep. The pain medicine made her drowsy, and she was ready to wake up to a new day and leave today in the past.

They drove back to Magnolia Hill.

Jenna dozed through most of the ride and woke to the flashing of the lights of utility trucks on the county road leading to her house. When they approached the area where the tornado had passed, Jenna flinched. They had to slow down for road crews still clearing the trees off the road and fixing the power lines.

"Looks like they moved your car port out of the way and pulled the tree trunk from your driveway," Cody said as they turned onto her property.

"I'm sorry, Cody," Jenna said. "I didn't mean to keep you up all night."

"I wouldn't have done it if I didn't want to."

"Actually, wait right here for a moment. I'll check on that tree before we go in," he said, then disappeared behind the house.

When he came back, she could tell something was wrong. He sat down in the driver's seat again. "Please don't tell me…"

"I hate to break this to you, but it looks worse than I had expected. You have a nice skylight and a hole in the side of the house above your window."

Jenna groaned. "Dang that old, rotten pine!" She wanted it removed for years and never had gotten around to it. Well, it was gone now.

"Looks like some folks chopped up the tree and put a tarp on your roof and the wall where your window was," he said, "but we won't know until daylight how bad it really is." He paused, then turned to her. "I can't leave you here by yourself. Why don't you stay at my house down the road, if it's still intact? We'll sort things out tomorrow. I'll postpone my appointments."

She wanted to tell him it wasn't necessary, but he had a

point. She had no power in the house, only half a roof, and one working arm. Besides, she couldn't wake up Beth in the middle of the night to take her in. She was tired, and all she wanted to do was sleep. She yawned into her uninjured hand. "Okay, let me go grab some fresh clothes, though."

He helped her out of the car and unlocked the door for her. Cody used his phone as a flashlight and held it for her as she gathered her overnight clothes and her hygiene items.

A few minutes later, Cody carried her bag, locked the door behind them, and they drove a mile down the road. After dodging more debris on the road, he turned into a long gravel driveway. "We're in luck. My house is still standing, by the looks of it."

His house was not as grand as she had thought it would be. At least, it didn't look so impressive in the dark. It was rather modest and about the size of her own house. She could make out some strange structures behind his home as the headlights shone on them but wasn't sure what to make of them.

"This is it." He came around, asked for her purse, then helped her out.

"Ouch," she winced. "I think my medicine is wearing off."

He supported her by her back. "We have all the time you need," he said as he walked her to his porch steps.

She was so tired that his supportive touch almost made her lean into him. *No, Jenna, he's a stranger*, she thought, and got all her strength together to walk up the steps on her own. Oh, how good it would feel, though, to have him carry her inside and put her on the bed, or sofa in this case, so she could sleep in his embrace. Shocked by her own thoughts, she stopped on the porch.

"Are you in pain? Do you need a break?" he asked with genuine concern on his face.

Thank goodness it was dark, or he would've seen her blush. It must be her meds making her hallucinate and think strange thoughts. "No, sorry. I'm good."

He unlocked the front door and switched his lights on. At least he tried to. "Sorry, my power is out, too," he said, and with his cell phone light walked her over to his couch. "Have a seat while I look for a flashlight."

Here she was on this stranger's couch in the dark. Her house was partially demolished, her car port was a goner, and she couldn't work in her shop. The impact of last night's events hit her like a solid punch in the gut, and there was nothing she could do right now but let the emotions flow. What was she going to do? Hot tears rolled down her face.

Cody came back with a large lantern-type flashlight that could illuminate the entire county. He then walked into the kitchen, rummaged around, and returned with a sandwich, a cup of water, and her pain meds, but she wasn't capable of caring right now.

He set the flashlight down on the dining room table and joined her on the couch. "You should eat something before you take your pain pill, so you won't get sick," he said, then noticed that she was crying. He gently wrapped his arm around her shoulder and carefully pulled her close. "Hey, hey. It's okay, Jenna. You're tired, and you've just been through a tornado. It'll all be better tomorrow."

"How, Dr. Walker?" she asked. How could it be all better?

"I honestly don't know, and it's Cody, remember?"

≈

*J*enna woke in the morning in what she assumed was Doc Walker's—no, Cody's— guest bedroom. A dull ache pulsed through her arm and her muscles screamed with the tiniest movement. She rolled onto her good side and pushed her way up into a sitting position. "Ouch, that hurts," she hissed more to herself. The aroma of coffee and breakfast hung in the air, but her stomach told her in no uncertain terms not to even think about eating. Besides, her to-do list today was long, and the sooner she got started on it, the better.

"Good morning, Jenna," Cody said, knocking lightly on the door frame. "May I come in?"

"Yes, of course," she said.

He entered the room with a tray of coffee, water, eggs, and sausage links. On the side, he had her bottle of medicine.

Now that he was wearing a t-shirt with his pajama bottoms, and the way he carried the tray, she could tell that he must work out. She turned her attention to her shoulder, so he wouldn't think that she was staring at him, which she was, but she didn't want to be obvious about it.

"The power's on again. Eat something first before you take your meds, or you'll most likely regret it."

"I already am."

He gave her a hurt look. "That's the new breakfast of champions, a secret recipe for aspiring ninja warriors."

"No, I didn't mean that. I'm just a bit nauseous." She glanced out of the bedroom window and saw the structures from when she first gotten to the house. "Wow, you're into cross-fit?"

He opened the blinds for her. "More into the ninja warrior stuff," he said. "It's a lot of fun and an incredible workout."

She smiled when she remembered playing on playground equipment not dissimilar to what Cody had set up on his land. "It looks like a playground for grown-ups."

He nodded. "That's what I had in mind. I'm toying with the idea of opening it up to the community, but there a lot of legalities to consider."

"I'd like to try one day." She pointed at her shoulder. "Once this is healed, of course."

"You do?"

"Why not?" She pushed her scrambled eggs around with her fork, then took a bite of the sausage. "I used to love those rings and bars as a kid." She didn't tell him she'd competed in gymnastics until her parents ran out of money, and that was the end of that.

"I think we can arrange that." His face became somber. "How are you feeling today?"

"Like I got picked up and dropped by a tornado." She laughed and took another bite. It was apparent that he didn't find her joke funny. "To be honest, I hurt all over."

"I figured you would," he said. "Once you take your pill, you'll probably want to nap a little more, and when you wake up, I'll be happy to take you to your house to inspect the damage."

"Don't you have patients to see?" she asked.

"I told Twyla to clear my schedule, so I'm free today," he said with a smile. "Then we can come back and tackle the insurance."

"Oh no. My shop!" She checked her phone. "Did Beth call?"

Cody shrugged his shoulders. "I didn't hear your phone ring. But I'll give you some privacy," he said. "I'm going to take a shower, and then I can take you to your house whenever you're ready to venture out there."

"Thanks," she said, then swallowed her pill.

"You're welcome," he replied with a smile and disappeared out of her room.

She dialed Beth's number. "Hey, how's the bakery?"

"Don't worry, we got everything covered. Clarissa is about to finish up the wedding cake and she decorated a couple of batches of cupcakes I baked earlier. She'll have to leave for her day job soon, but she was a big help this morning."

Jenna took a sigh of relief. "Thank you, Beth. I owe you both so much."

"That's not all," her friend continued. "I called Willow last night to offer her the job, and she came in this morning. She said it's okay if you want to do the official paperwork later. You rest, and we'll talk when you're up to it. We'll make do in the meantime. How's your house?"

"I had that old tree fall onto my roof. And when I came home last night, somebody had already cut up the tree and tarped the roof and the side of the house for me." She wasn't even going to tell her where she was now and what she was doing. Next thing she'd know, it would be all over town. Even though she trusted Beth, she didn't want to risk it. "I'll have to make a lot of calls today, but I'll be in later if I can. Hey, if you ladies have any questions at all, call me, okay?"

"I promise. Like I said, take care of your things first,

and we'll keep the bakery going in the meantime. Our cupcakes may not be as pretty, but they'll do in a pinch."

"Thanks, Beth. What would I do without you?" she asked. "Talk to you later, okay?" They ended the call, and Jenna put her phone back on the nightstand.

With her stomach less queasy, she took a few more bites of her now cold breakfast and a sip of coffee, then set the tray aside and laid back down. Who would've thought that Cody would open his home to a stranger like her? This just showed her how wrong she had been about him. On the other hand, he really had been a jerk the other day. The worst part was that the glimpses she'd seen from the real Cody were ones of a kind and caring man who'd do anything for anyone—even her, a small-town girl from Magnolia Hill, Georgia. Okay, there was a worse part than that. Every time they had accidentally touched last night, she wanted to fall into his arms. She did when she bawled her eyes out, but she'd rather forget about that—the embarrassing bawling part, not the burying her face in his chest part. *Oh, these pain meds must cloud her mind*, she thought, because she would never open up to a stranger like that. And why was she so determined to get close to him?

She closed her eyes. No, she had to keep her mind straight. This was not her talking.

The reality was that he came into the shop acting crazy and demanding outrageous things like keeping the cake smell down. Hello? This was a bakery. Then this rich-boy car thing never boded well in relationships. Just because his house was modest, his choice of car said a lot about him. Twice before she had fallen for those corporate types, and twice she got her feelings hurt pretty badly. She couldn't let that happen again, even though his outside appearance was at odds with the character traits he showed her in the last twelve hours. Still, that outburst…

Jenna couldn't and shouldn't risk falling in love with him, no matter how nice he was. He was still the enemy. She swore she would not have another lapse of judgment.

CHAPTER EIGHT

*C*ody opened his car door for Jenna and helped her in. He winced at the sight of his cracked windshield and the couple of dents, but he'd get that fixed soon. Jenna came first. "I hope that tree didn't cause too much structural damage to your house, although it didn't look good last night."

"Me, too," Jenna said. "Thank goodness for insurance, even though paying for my deductible will hurt."

Cody drove them down the road, and as they got closer to her house, a path of twisted trees was proof that the tornado tore through the area yesterday evening. His chest tightened with the realization of how lucky she was she didn't get killed.

Jenna's mouth gaped as they drove by the destruction. "This is so surreal," she said. "I don't know if I would've survived if…" she trailed off.

"You must have a guardian angel," he said. And he meant it.

Jenna nodded. "I think I do."

The white upside-down carport on the side of the road told him he was at the right house. They turned off the road and onto her property. Cody tried to be careful about not hitting too many potholes but couldn't avoid them all.

With each bump, Jenna let out a soft hiss.

"I'm sorry. I didn't mean to cause more pain than necessary," he said.

"That's okay," she said. "I've been planning on getting my driveway paved, but that's another project I couldn't afford yet."

Cody pulled up behind her car and turned off the engine. From the front, the house didn't look too bad. Granted, the carport was still on the side of the road, and the corner of the house where the tornado had tossed her was still cluttered. But it amazed him that her house wasn't leveled. If the twister would've shifted a couple more yards east, they wouldn't be sitting on her driveway about to assess the damage the tornado had caused.

"The side of the house looks empty without my carport," she said.

"But your SUV is still there," he replied with a smile. Cody got out of his car and helped her out.

She walked around her car to inspect it, letting her fingers graze over the large cupcake decal on the side of the vehicle. "Amazing. Not even a dent."

Cody smiled. "You really lucked out." He nodded at his car. "Mine took a slight beating."

They walked to the back of the house.

Jenna cupped her mouth with her good hand. "Oh, no!"

Someone had pulled the tree off her house and cut it into large logs, but tarps covering the roof and the side of the house meant there was significant damage.

"Let me get your overnight bag and purse, and we can go check the damage from the inside," Cody suggested.

"Thanks," she said, walking with him to the side entrance of the house.

As he walked back to the car, Cody's chest tightened with guilt. His outburst the first time they met was uncalled for, especially now that he was getting to know her. His own addiction to sweets and comfort food had clouded his judgement, and he hadn't seen her as a person. Now he saw her as the kind and hard-working woman she was, and he felt like a jerk for behaving the way he did. He grabbed her purse and bag from the backseat of his car and headed back to meet her by the side-door where she was waiting for him. He held her purse open for her. "Can you find your keys? I didn't want to search through your belongings." Warmth spread to his face.

"It's fine," she said as she hovered over her purse and pulled out her keys. "I don't think there's anything dangerous in there that might bite your fingers off," she said with a grin. She unlocked the door and led him through the laundry room into the kitchen.

Cody noticed a piece of paper with a note on the kitchen counter. "I think your helpers might have left you a note." He pointed at the letter.

Jenna picked it up and read it out loud. "Jenna, I hope you're feeling better when you find this note. We've pulled the tree off your house and covered the hole in the roof and the wall to prevent further damage. If you want, we'll be back this weekend to finish cutting up the tree for firewood. We checked your wiring, and it's safe, but you may want to keep out of your bedroom until the damage is fixed. Let us know if there's anything else we can do for you. We started a collection to help with deductibles and such, and your spare key is back under the planter. Best, Chief Jordan at Station 1."

She put the letter down and smiled at him with teary eyes.

Cody was about to joke about Station 1 being the only fire station in town, but he could tell she was trying not to fall apart. Seeing her so vulnerable made his insides turn to mush. Not sure what else to do, he took a step toward her and gently embraced her, careful not to touch her shoulder. "I can tell the people in this town care a great deal about you."

She snuggled up to his chest, wiping a tear from her cheek with her good hand. "We all are one big family. We help each other out when someone is in need. That's what we do here."

He caressed her good shoulder. "Like I said, you're very lucky."

Jenna lifted her head. Their eyes met. "I…"

Cody didn't know what to do. They were treading on dangerous territory. How she landed in his arms again was beyond him. Why did everything have to be so complicated?

Jenna inhaled, then stepped back, wiping a last stray tear off her face and shaking her head. "I'm sorry. I didn't mean to…"

The awkwardness that hung in the air was almost tangible. "Let's check your bedroom for damage," he tried to distract.

"Right," Jenna said and took the lead to the back of the house.

The smell of damp, fresh tree greeted them. The hole

in the roof and smashed-in area above the window looked worse than he had expected. "Look, Jenna, if you need a place to stay until the insurance sends out someone to fix your bedroom, I have that empty guest room available for you."

"Thanks, Cody, but I don't think that's a good idea. Besides, I won't let this tornado beat me down. I'll be okay."

He had to agree and admired her strength. Having her stay with him probably wasn't appropriate, especially since they still had this elephant standing between them in the room.

"If you don't mind, can you drop me off at the bakery after I call the insurance company? I want to check on how things are going with my two new employees. That way you can go back to your practice."

"I can give you a ride home later, too, if you want," he offered, hoping to spend some more time with her.

"Thank you, Cody, but Beth can give me a ride and help me get settled into my spare bedroom."

Maybe it's for the better, he thought, and ignored the pinch of disappointment. Cody knew they were not okay. Instead of feeling sorry for himself, his time would be better spent on catching up on patient charts and maybe throwing some darts at the Sappy Pine afterwards. It's Friday night, after all.

∼

"Thank you again for everything," Jenna said to Cody as they parted ways at the parking spot in front of her shop.

"The offer still stands. Call me if you need anything at all, day or night, okay?"

"Will do. But now I have to check in on my staff." She waved at him and rushed toward the door. She could see Beth watching through the window and pointed at her as to give her a warning.

Cody rushed past her and opened the door with a smile. "Allow me."

"Well, thank you," she said, flattered at his southern manners. It was a plus in her book, but she needed many more pluses to make up for that big fat minus over a week ago, and only time would tell.

"Bye, Jenna!" he said, then moved his car to his usual parking spot across the street.

Jenna looked back at him and noticed the curtain of the window facing the street move. *Twyla,* she thought, and smiled.

"Oh my gosh, Jenna. I don't know where to start." Beth ambushed her. "Are you okay? Did I just see you being friendly with Doc Walker?" Her facial expression turned into a frown.

"Yes, I'm fine. And he's just being nice," Jenna replied.

"I didn't think he was capable of that. Why are you even talking to him?" she asked, her face perplexed.

"It's a long story, Beth, and I'll catch you up later."

Willow approached them with a bottle of glass cleaner and a few paper towels in hand. "Hello, Ms. Wilson, and thank you so much for letting me work here."

"Hi, Willow. Welcome, and please call me Jenna. I should thank you for starting at such short notice. Beth has told me how quickly you caught on and how big of a help you've been today."

Willow blushed a little, which was a perfect contrast to her dark blue hair. "Thank you. I really don't mind."

"Well, we're happy to have you," Jenna said. "If you want, you can take the rest of the afternoon off. You've done a lot of work already today, and Friday afternoons are usually slow, anyway. We can start your paperwork Monday."

"Yes, ma'am. Thank you," Willow said. She put away the cleaner and paper towels and grabbed her backpack. "Have a nice weekend, Ms. Jenna and Ms. Beth."

Beth didn't waste any time. "So, tell me about your house," Beth said. "I really didn't expect you here today."

"It's a mess. There's a large hole in the roof, and my bedroom is full of twigs and leaves," Jenna said. "I called insurance, and I'm meeting the adjuster at noon tomorrow. There's not much more I could do at home today, so I asked Cody to give me a ride to the shop."

"You can't work with your arm in the sling!" Beth said, her arms propped on her hips.

"I may not be able to lift anything, but I can teach," Jenna said. "I can talk you through a few recipes. Just because I'm hurt doesn't mean I'm useless. I still have a brain, just not both my arms." At least being at work beat sitting at the house and doing nothing but worrying about the survival of the bakery—and thinking of Cody.

Beth's eyes lit up.

"How did Clarissa work out this morning?" Jenna asked.

Beth shifted uncomfortably. "Well, how should I say it? She was Clarissa—always happy to take charge and orchestrate," Beth said. "Maybe you were right, and it was a mistake to ask her to fill in."

Jenna knew Clarissa would be a problem, but she was also an excellent baker. She'd have to call her and diffuse the situation before it could get out of hand. Right now, she didn't have a choice. Beth wasn't ready to bake full force yet, and Willow probably needed a few more days to get worked in. "I'll talk to her."

"Thanks. Now that that's out of the way, I want to know about Doc Walker," Beth said, her elbows resting on the counter, waiting for the juicy details.

As if on cue, the doorbells chimed, and Anna entered the shop. "What are you doing at work, Jenna? Aren't you supposed to be home resting?"

Jenna rolled her eyes.

"Well, good timing, Anna, because our friend here was about to tell me how come she's suddenly friendly with Doc Walker across the street."

"Oh?" Anna raised both hands to her cheeks in mock surprise. "Come to think of it, wasn't there a moment between the two of you before we took you into the ambulance?"

"A moment?" Beth asked. "What's going on here? Isn't the new doc our number one enemy?"

"What was it you come in for, Anna?" Jenna deflected.

"Mom sent me to pick up some cupcakes for her knitting class at the Spinning Yarns shop tonight. The ladies love them, and we love to keep them happy. But the cupcakes can wait. What were you about to say about the new doc?"

"I wasn't going to say anything," Jenna replied. Beth

had a point. He was her enemy. She had to stay smart and not give into her emotions. Her shop depended on it.

"Come on, Jenna. Tell us what happened," Beth coaxed.

"We're all ears," Anna added.

Jenna closed her eyes. Her mind raced in a tug-of-war between thoughts of Cody caring for her and him threatening to shut down her business. They were her friends—the only people in the world she could trust with her feelings. She had to confide in someone, or she risked losing her mind. "Promise me not to tell a soul?"

"I promise," Beth said. "My lips are sealed."

"Cross my heart and hope to die," Anna said.

"Okay, so here's what happened," Jenna began.

CHAPTER NINE

ody sat in his office chair. He heard Beth and Jenna laughing as they closed the bakery up, then watched them drive off. He wished it would've been him taking her back to her house just for the company—or better yet, his house—but he knew it wasn't to be. Instead, he skipped his evening workout and headed over to the Sappy Pine. Not that he liked to hang around people after work, but he needed to distract himself from the events of the last twenty-four hours.

He closed the last record on his desk, grabbed his coat, and walked a block down the street to the bar.

Cody opened the door and found a spot to sit in a booth.

A waitress approached his table. "What can I get you, Doc?" she asked.

A beer would've been nice, but he reconsidered when he reminded himself of the carb count. Maybe he'd have one for a special occasion one day, but today was not one of those. Besides, he had to be a role model for his patients. "Just an unsweetened iced tea with a lemon," he said instead.

"Do you need a menu?" she asked.

"I'm good for now. Maybe later." He gave her a quick smile, then let it drop again when she turned away from him.

As he sat and waited for his beverage, he drummed his fingers on the marred wooden table. Some lovebirds had carved a heart and the initials JM & AW on the tabletop, close to where it met the wall. Judging by the dark outline, it had been there for a long time. He wondered if JM & AW were still madly in love. *Must be nice to have someone you can't even think of spending a minute apart from,* he thought. Maybe one day he'd be so lucky. He very much liked the idea of having someone to share the highs and lows of life with. All these years, he had spent most of his time working and saving the world, and dating was the last thing on his mind. Besides, who would want to be in a relationship with someone who worked long hours like he did and came home exhausted? That special someone who would be in his life would not deserve a boring guy like him.

The waitress returned with his tea, set it on a napkin to catch the sweat off the glass, and handed him a straw. "Here ya go, hun. Uh, Doc."

"Thank you," he said and squeezed the lemon into his tea. He knew lemon was not the most sanitary additive—who knew how long this slice had been sitting out and how many people had touched it—but since he couldn't have a beer, he'd take the risk.

The door to the bar opened again, and Sean entered, followed by another man who looked vaguely familiar.

Sean, with a slight limp, and the other guy walked toward his table.

"Evenin', Cody," he said. "Mind if we sit here, or are you expecting company?"

Cody gestured for them to have a seat. "Nah, I just wasn't ready to head home yet," he admitted.

"I don't blame you." Sean scooted to the inside of the booth. "Cody, have you met my buddy Jason Morrison yet?"

"I don't believe I have, although you do look familiar," Cody said and extended his hand, noticing a small pink scar on Jason's forehead that couldn't be too old. "Cody Walker. I took over Doc Porter's practice. Are you a patient of mine?"

Jason shook his hand. "I am; I just hadn't been in to see you yet."

"I swear I've seen you before." It bothered Cody he couldn't pin down where he knew this man from.

Sean signaled the waitress to bring them two beers. "He's the weatherman on Channel 12."

"Chief Meteorologist," he corrected Sean, "which means I do not only forecast the weather, I also get the wonderful pleasure of having to deal with the typical staffing issues of my team."

So that's where he'd seen him before. "Well, it's good to meet you."

Sean laughed.

"What's so funny?" Jason asked.

"You should watch the video when Jason was covering Hurricane Gerard that hit Tybee Island in August."

Jason scowled at his friend. "Don't listen to him, Cody."

Sean ignored him and continued. "Look up meteorologist hit by flying plywood on your phone. It's hilarious and went viral worldwide."

Jason blushed. "It wasn't that funny," he said.

The waitress dropped off the two bottles of beer and two glasses.

"Oh, sure it was," Sean said.

"I might check it out later," Cody said. Feeling sorry for that poor guy trying to hide his embarrassment, he changed the subject. "How's your foot, Sean?"

"Better today," he said. "Still sore as all get out, but I've been through worse."

Both Sean and Jason pulled out their buzzing cell phones from their pockets.

"Kids," Jason said, holding up his phone.

"Grady is asking to go to the movies tonight," Sean said. He looked up at Cody. "Grady is my teenage son."

"And this is my daughter Ashleigh asking if she and Sarah can go to the movies with Grady," Jason said, pointing at his phone. "Anna must be busy at work. They usually ask her first. You might know my fiancé, Anna. She's a paramedic with the fire department."

"Dark hair?" Cody asked.

Jason nodded. "Yep."

Of course she was, he thought. "I met her after the tornado transplanted Jenna's carport," Cody replied, not wanting to mention her cool demeanor toward him.

"Jenna got lucky," Jason added, pouring his beer into the glass in front of him and taking a sip. "Good news is that she only dislocated her shoulder and got a big goose-egg on her noggin."

"How did you know?" Cody asked.

"Small town," Jason replied with a grin. "There are no secrets here."

Cody smiled and shook his head. He forgot what it was like to live in a community where everybody knew each other and also knew everybody's business.

"So, Jenna told Beth, who told me when she picked up a late lunch at Mamaw's, that you have a ninja playground in your backyard," Sean said.

Cody nodded. He remembered that Jenna wanted to try it out after her shoulder had healed. All this talk about his distant neighbor made him wondered how she was doing. Maybe he should call her to make sure she was okay in her battered house.

"Cody?" Sean said, and both men looked at him in anticipation of an answer.

"Yes, I do."

"Well, when can we come over and put it to use?" Jason asked, rubbing his hands together as if someone just handed him a Christmas gift.

"This weekend is going to be nice if you both want to come over." He frowned. "Sean, you'll have to take it easy with your foot, though, for now."

"I will." Sean patted his slightly protruding belly. "Even if I tried, my body won't let me overdo it. It's been a while since I've done some real exercising, if you know what I mean."

"I can't believe we have someone with cool-guy stuff in town," Jason said, still with that grin plastered on his face.

Cody smiled. He wasn't ready to share his plans yet of eventually opening his Ninja Course as a side business. Not until he had his ducks in a row.

"So, Anna told me that Jenna likes you," Jason said. "But don't tell her I told you. This is just between us guys. I've got to keep the peace at home."

Cody almost choked on his tea. He didn't see that one coming.

"So, what's the deal?" Sean asked. "I saw the look between you two when Anna put her in the ambulance."

"Isn't there a rule about doctors dating their patients?" Jason added.

"It's nothing," Cody said.

"Sure," Sean taunted, drawing out the word.

"No, really, Sean." Cody wasn't sure if he could trust these two guys with opening up, but they were his closest friends, if he could even call it that, he had in this town. He was the new guy—the outsider. Maybe if he kept specifics out, he could talk about the pickle he got himself into. "This is between us?"

"Just between us," Sean promised.

"To answer your question, Jason," Cody continued, "yes, there is an ethical rule that physicians can't date their patients."

The guys leaned back into their seat.

"That would be a problem," Jason said, cupping his chin.

"Not really," Cody added, "because she's not my patient."

Sean squinted his eyes. "What do you mean? Everyone in Magnolia Hill saw Doc Porter."

Cody sighed. "There's a conflict of interest—a significant one." When neither one responded, he continued. "I am the Magnolia Hill's family physician. My job is to keep my patients healthy or help them get better."

"Okay," Jason said. "So why would dating Jenna be a problem then?"

"She makes cupcakes, and no doubt very delicious ones," Cody said. "I have diabetic patients going straight across the street for cupcakes after they promised to take sugar and high-carb processed foods out of their diet."

"Oh, that's a bummer," Sean said. "I can understand why."

Jason took a sip of his beer. "If it makes you feel better, Anna's mom, Maggie, says she can't have sweet stuff anymore. Anna started eating low carb too, to support her, but every once in a while, she sneaks a cupcake."

"See what I mean?" Cody said. "Diabetics can't metabolize sugar well. When they keep over-indulging these frankenfoods, their body can only do so much damage control. Next thing you know, they develop neuropathy, kidney problems, blindness, and a host of other issues."

"And you're saying it's Jenna's fault?" Sean asked.

"This goes much deeper, but it's part of the problem. I might at one point have been a little hot-headed, went to her shop, and told her she's technically killing the people of this town." He watched the two men shift in their seats and avoid eye contact with him. Cody knew he had overstepped a boundary. It was a bed he had made for himself, but he also had a duty to save his patients. Do no harm was the oath he took as a physician. But was he doing more harm by being so passionate about saving people?

"I see," Jason said. "Jenna is as sweet as they come, no pun intended. She's good people and she would never do that."

Cody put his head in his hands. "I know that now, but I'm afraid that I messed everything up that first time we met. I can tell that she's just being nice, but there's still that dark cloud hovering above us, and until that's resolved, this can never work. And I don't know where to begin with making things right with her."

Jason took the last gulp of his beer. "That's easy. Relationships are all about compromises. Trust me, I know. Can't you both find a way to meet in the middle?"

~

*I*t was a cool and early morning when Jenna drove herself one-handedly to the shop. She was running late. Five minutes into her usual morning routine, she had realized that she wouldn't make it to the bakery before Beth and Clarissa arrived. Jenna was grateful for the mayor's wife agreeing to help Beth decorate cupcakes for the morning rush before her Chamber job. Without her help, the bakery would run out of inventory halfway through each day.

She checked the time on her dash and gently pushed the gas pedal down a bit more. Sean wouldn't pull her over for speeding and not signaling with her bad arm. Or would he?

With a jerky right-hand turn, she pulled into a vacant parking space on Main Street a few spaces away from her shop entrance.

"Good morning, Beth," she greeted her friend.

"Mornin' Jenna," Beth said as she moved a batch of fresh cupcakes onto a cooling rack. "What did the insurance adjuster say about your carport and your skylight?"

"It'll cost a lot, but they'll try to get a contractor out to work on the repairs this week," Jenna said as she struggled to take off her coat with her one good arm.

"That's awesome news," Beth said, coming to Jenna's aid.

"Beth, I need the next batch of cupcakes. Now," a shrill voice demanded from the pantry area, becoming louder as the rotund woman with full make-up came closer. "I told you I only have two hours before I have to head out to the Chamber. If I would've known you're that slow, I could've baked them myself. This is unsatis…" She trailed off as she caught sight of Jenna. "Oh, hello, Jenna," Clarissa said with a smile.

"See what I mean?" Beth mumbled under her breath.

Jenna walked over to Clarissa and hooked her arm under the woman's. "Good morning, Clarissa. May I have a word?"

"I don't see why, but yes," Clarissa answered.

Jenna sent up a silent prayer that Clarissa wouldn't misunderstand what she was about to say. She led her to the table in the kitchen's back corner. "Please, have a seat."

After Beth disappeared out of the kitchen to the front of the bakery, Jenna turned to Clarissa. Her heart was pounding. Jenna had to tread lightly as to not get on her bad side. The woman was a force of her own, and if she approached this the wrong way, Clarissa could turn the entire town against her. She'd seen her do it when the then single Ms. Fisher batted her eyes at the mayor during the fall festival ten years ago. They still didn't speak to this day, and it took Ms. Fisher three years to beat her reputation as a home wrecker. That's all Jenna needed, especially after the Cody incident.

"What's this about? Are you not happy with the cupcakes?" she asked. "Did I top them with too much icing?"

Here goes nothing, Jenna thought. "No, the cupcakes are wonderful." She leaned forward and rested her good arm on the table. "Please don't take this the wrong way, but we are like a family in this business. The Cherry on Top Cupcake Shop is a cheerful and happy place, and we all work together as a team."

"What does this have to do with me? I'm friends with everyone in this town," Clarissa asked.

"Well," Jenna was careful to choose her words wisely. "You're strong, confident, and successful, which are noble traits, but it can come across as intimidating or overpowering for some people."

The woman across from her huffed. "I'm not overpowering! I just get things done. If you ask me, I'm doing you a favor. We're getting a lot done in record time."

Jenna cringed. That didn't go as well as she had expected. Actually, it went exactly how she thought this conversation would go. "Clarissa, I'm so glad you are here to help, but…"

Clarissa stood, took off her apron, and tossed it on the table. "If you don't want me here, then fine. I'm happy to get out of your way."

Jenna noticed Clarissa's eyes well up. She stood and held out her good hand. "No, Clarissa. I want you here. I need you here. Don't go."

"It's too late," the mayor's wife said. "Some words cannot be unsaid. I know when I'm not wanted." The woman turned and walked out.

"Clarissa!"

CHAPTER TEN

Cupcakes flew off the shelves all morning long, and while Willow was holding down the fort in the shop area, Jenna was talking Beth through a more complicated and delicate recipe—the I Dream of Chocolate Lava Cupcake—a local favorite among their customers. Anna had called it the Death by Chocolate cupcake the other day.

Death by chocolate. Her chest tightened with the memory of Cody accusing her of killing her patients. Was he still trying to shut her down? Maybe he was only this nice to her now because she got injured. She didn't know what to make of him. Jenna had seen the softer side of Cody, but her spidey senses kicked in when she thought of that first confrontation. She so much wanted him to be the same man who helped her the day of the tornado, but their business interests were completely at odds. Life wasn't fair. All her friends had found their soulmates, and she even took some credit for pushing them in the right directions. Her intuition for matching the perfect couples worked like a charm—for anyone but herself.

The front door chimed, and a moment later, Willow poked her head with her hair in high-set Princess Leia buns through the kitchen doorway. "Jenna, Doc Walker is here and needs to talk to you."

Jenna had a chill run down her spine. Was he having another episode? Reluctantly, she wiped her good hand on her apron, took a deep breath, and headed into the shop.

Cody smiled at her from the other side of the counter. "Hi."

She relaxed. At least he didn't look like he was blowing up on her again. "Hi." She noticed him holding a covered disposable baking pan.

He set the pan on the counter. "How's your shoulder?"

"It's getting better. I have a follow-up appointment with my doctor in Richmond Hill on Wednesday."

He his head toward the street. "I saw your SUV parked out front. Don't tell me you drove yourself."

She shrugged. "I used to drive with a hamburger in one hand, a drink in the other, and steer with my knees. I'm good."

"Not that it's my business," Beth interjected, "but I did offer to pick her up this morning, and she refused." She shook her head. "If you ask me, this woman is stubborn as a mule."

Jenna pointed at the baking dish. "What's this?"

He lifted his left eyebrow. "A peace offering."

"Let's see!" Jenna said, trying to uncover the pan. "Can you help me lift the foil off?"

He uncurled the aluminum from the sides of the pan and lifted it off with just a touch of resistance. Inside the baking pan were almost a dozen of white cupcakes in dotted cupcake paper squished into a corner. Half the cream-colored icing stuck to the foil. "Oh, no. Excuse the minor frosting accident," he said with a slight blush.

"You made cupcakes?" she asked.

Cody nodded. "I did. I'm not a baker by any means, but try them." He nodded at Willow and Beth. "You ladies, too."

Reluctantly, Jenna picked up one of the cupcakes. "These aren't poisoned, are they?"

"Of course not," he said with a mock-hurt facial expression, and picked one up for himself.

She peeled back the paper. Hopefully, they tasted better than they looked. Jenna hesitated, then took her first bite. "Hmm, not half-bad." She was pleasantly surprised how fluffy and flavorful it was.

"So, you like them?" he asked.

"The presentation might need some work, but for starters, these are actually pretty good."

He smiled. "I know that these do not measure up to your cupcakes, but they are low carb."

"So, what are you proposing?" she asked.

"First, I wanted to apologize for my behavior again the last time I blew my top." He flushed a little. "It was uncalled for, and I overreacted."

Did he really just apologize to her and admit he was wrong? "Thank you, I appreciate that."

"I also spent all weekend trying to find a solution to this cupcake versus patient dilemma we seem to have. There has to be a way to keep us both happy, and I think I figured it out."

"You bake cupcakes for your patients?" Beth asked.

Jenna shook her head. "I know my customers, but if they had the choice…" She looked down at his misshapen cupcakes.

"Don't you see, Jenna, we can refine these cupcakes to make them look as appetizing as yours. You could develop a line of diabetic-friendly, low-carb cupcakes and offer them here. That way my patients have an alternative we all could live with."

Willow nodded her head. "I like it—a line of doctor-approved treats."

"I think we should try it," Beth said to her friend.

"Well, I don't know." She'd have to buy all kinds of exotic ingredients, and she was already going to be a little tighter on money with both Willow and Clarissa working for her, at least for the time being.

"Oh, come on Jenna," Beth tried again to convince her. "They are really good."

"And I promise to send a bunch of my patients back to you," Cody added.

"What's in them?" she asked.

He looked up at the ceiling as if trying to remember. "Almond flour, coconut flour, psyllium husk, eggs, butter, and instead of sugar, I've used a monk fruit and erythritol mix. It doesn't have that cooling effect or bitter taste like some low-carb sweeteners, and it doesn't affect blood sugar levels."

Jenna frowned. "I'd have to order a lot of special ingredients, and the cost…"

Cody shook his head. "Those ingredients are commonly available nowadays and not as expensive as you think. You could charge a little extra for the low-carb cupcakes to make up for it."

Jenna tightened her lips. "They need work."

"Does that mean you'll give it a go?" he asked.

"Not yet," she said, "but I'll tell you what. Grab us a burger from Mamaw's Friday after I close up shop, bring a good supply of your cupcake ingredients, and be prepared to do some baking. We'll do some fine-tuning of the recipe."

Cody high-fived Beth, who stood next to him. "Thank you, Jenna. I'll be there and bring whatever you want."

~

"Willow, Beth, will you be okay for about half an hour while I walk over to the Chamber to talk to Clarissa?" Jenna asked, hanging her apron on a hook.

"Why?" Beth said. "Working with her the last couple of mornings reminded me why I can't stand that woman. I should've never suggested that she should help us at the bakery. That was all my fault. And to be honest, I'm glad she walked out, regardless of how good her baking is."

"Now, Beth," Jenna said and laid a hand on her shoulder. "I know you better than that. Clarissa is going through some hard times. You told me so yourself."

"That obviously was a lapse of judgment on my part, which I now regret," Beth said.

"I know she can be," Jenna paused for a moment to choose the right word, "loud and blunt."

"And bossy," Willow added.

"Yes, and bossy," Jenna said. "But we are in a pickle. Until my shoulder is healed, I can only do so much work in the kitchen. We need her help for at least another week or two to keep up with the demand. Trust me, I thought about this all morning."

"I don't know if this is a good idea to bring her back," Beth said. "Two weeks with Clarissa is a long time. At this point, one morning is too long to handle."

"Let me worry about this. I may have figured out a solution that could work for all of us," Jenna said.

"Okay, you're the boss, even though I'm not convinced," Beth said. "I better get another batch of cupcakes started. Good luck with Clarissa, I guess?"

"Don't worry. It'll be fine," Jenna said. "I'll be back soon."

The noon sun warmed Jenna's face as she walked down Main Street to the Chamber building. Her shoulder ached, but the pain was mild compared to the day after the tornado. Hopefully, she could get that arm out of her sling soon. She felt useless not being able to work much. All she could do was stand there and teach Beth or help Willow with customers. Jenna took pride in her independence, but since the tornado, that independence was out of the window. She had never been one to ask for help, but now, she had to do it. Worse yet, she had to ask Clarissa to consider coming back.

Jenna opened one of the heavy wooden doors to the Chamber and walked into the foyer. She could hear Clarissa's shrill voice from her office down the hall. Dread filled her gut, but she had to do it. She had no choice. A strong whiff of perfume greeted her. With a soft knock on the open door, she stepped into Clarissa's office. "May I come in?" she asked, her heart beating harder than it should. Why she was intimidated by the mayor's wife was beyond her.

"Might as well," she said. "But I'm not sure why you're here. I'm not coming back. Sorry, you wasted your time."

"If you could give me just a few minutes anyway?" Jenna asked. "Please?"

Clarissa's facial expression softened. "Okay, go ahead, since you're already here."

"Thank you," Jenna said, relieved she didn't kick her out right away. "First, I want you to know how thankful I am that you've helped with the wedding cake after the tornado."

"Of course, the bride was my best friend's daughter," Clarissa said in a flat tone.

"I also want you to know that I very much appreciate you coming in early in the mornings to help with the cupcakes before your day job. This has to be hard for you, and I don't even know how to thank you. Without your help, we would run out of cupcakes by noon every day."

Clarissa leaned back in her overstuffed office chair. "Well, I have to admit, since you've opened your bakery, you've become one of Magnolia Hill's most favorite businesses, next to the Spinning Yarns Craft Shop, of course. As a popular Chamber member, it wouldn't look good for our organization if you'd offer inferior products, even if temporary. That's the only reason I agreed to help."

"So you see why we need you to come back," Jenna ventured. "Just until my shoulder heals well enough to where I can bake again."

"Yes. But I also know when I'm not wanted," Clarissa said. "You made that clear this morning. So, the answer is still no."

This was going nowhere. Jenna had to change tactics.

"Look, Clarissa, you've got the gift of baking wonderful pies and pastries, and your cake decorating skills are out of this world. You're a natural. We only need you for a couple of hours in the mornings. How about if Beth, Willow, and I will get the bulk of the cupcakes baked and icing made in the afternoon, and in the mornings, you can focus on your decorating magic and create these beautiful cupcakes? We'll even section off a workspace for you so you can focus better." *And it would keep you and Beth out of each other's hair,* Jenna thought.

The woman blushed. "Well, thank you for the compliment, Jenna. And a separate workspace would make my job easier. It would certainly help having the cakes and icing ready, so I won't have to wait on Beth all morning. But I don't know. This getting up early business is wearing on me."

"Give me two weeks?" Jenna leaned forward and whispered, "This is between us, but I know you're going through a rough patch and need some extra cash. I can't offer much, but it'll help. It's a win for both of us."

Clarissa's face took on a deep shade of red behind the heavy make-up. "You're right. But I'd appreciate it if you could keep my family's financial difficulties between the two of us."

"So, that means you're coming back?" Jenna asked, her voice letting out a little squeak at the end.

"Yes. I think I can handle two more weeks," Clarissa said.

Deep inside, Jenna jumped with joy. She had tamed the lion—at least for now. "I'll see you tomorrow morning, then?"

"I'll be there."

Jenna left the Chamber with almost a skip in her step. She had the help. The only challenge was to keep Clarissa and Beth busy and separated in the kitchen. *It was only two weeks*, she tried to tell herself.

CHAPTER ELEVEN

*W*ith his car loaded full of groceries and a passenger seat occupied by Mamaw's takeout boxes and drinks, he parked in front of the Cherry on Top Cupcake Shop. His heart was beating faster than he was used to, and a fleeting fear of another heart attack sent him into panic mode. He felt for his pulse and checked his smart watch. 106 beats per minute. Too fast, considering he wasn't doing anything strenuous.

Despite the panic spreading from his chest to his limbs and head, Cody relaxed into his seat. *It's not your heart,* he told himself. *This wave will pass in a few minutes and you'll be fine.* He inhaled, held his breath, then exhaled. Inhaled, held his breath, and exhaled again. Just when his heartbeat settled down, he noticed Jenna standing behind the shop door. She unlocked it to let him in.

He had waited all week for a chance to see her and work on his low-carb cupcakes with her. His worst fear was that he would mess things up with her again.

A few palpitations later, he closed his eyes, took a final

deep breath, and grabbed the food boxes from the passenger seat.

"Hi," she greeted him.

"Hi," he said. "As promised, I brought dinner."

"Thank you. I can take the food in if you want to get the groceries," she said, holding out her good arm. "Cody, you're shaking. Are you okay?"

"No worries, I'm fine. Probably just too much coffee at the practice today," he said, handing her the bag with the takeout boxes. As she took the food from him, he noticed that the scrapes on her skin were healing, and she wasn't wearing her sling, but was still cautious about moving her injured arm. "How's your shoulder?"

"It's getting better. My doctor said I'm healing nicely, and I can try keeping it off. It's still really sore, and I'm learning what I can and cannot do yet."

His doctor training kicked in. "What medication are you on? When do you start physical therapy?"

She laughed. "Do I detect a hint of jealousy? He's a good doctor, and yes, he already has me doing some exercises to get my mobility back. Physical therapy starts next week." Jenna nodded down at the boxes she was holding. "If you don't mind, I'm going to put these in the kitchen now. I'm starving!"

"Sorry," he said. "I got carried away. I'll grab the groceries and drinks and then join you for dinner."

Cody grabbed the bags of almond flour, the monk fruit sweetener, and the other ingredients he had purchased from one of the larger grocery stores in Savannah. Somehow, he managed to open the glass door to the bakery with one finger. "Thank you, ninja training," he whispered, then squeezed through the opening before it closed on him again.

"Just set all the stuff down on the counter by the mixer."

Cody saw something that resembled something like a giant kitchen aide and dropped the bags next to it.

By the time he had carried in the last bag, she had already set out their takeout boxes, arranged their napkins, ketchup, and mayo packets neatly on the table in the back of the kitchen, and was waving him over to join her.

He rubbed his hands together, sat down, and opened the box with his name written on it. "Rub-a-dub-dub, let's eat some grub!" he said.

Jenna smiled, and it warmed his heart.

"My mom used to say that when I was a kid," she said, opening her takeout box. "I love burgers from Mamaw's. The fries are just the perfect thickness and are crunchy on the outside and soft in the inside—just the way I like them." She demonstrated the point by picking up one of her fries and taking a bite.

"Looks delicious," Cody said and opened his box.

She stopped eating her fry and stared at his food instead.

He felt the blood rushing to his face. "It's low carb." Not that he had to justify his food choices, but by the look on her face, an explanation would be best. "I am a type 2 diabetic," he said. "In remission."

"You? I'm sorry to hear that, but I'm confused. You're eating a bun-less double half pound burger with cheese and mayo?"

Cody smiled. "I admit, the ingredients of the commercial mayo aren't the best. I usually make my own at home."

"But all the fat?" she asked. "Doesn't it clog your arteries?"

"The fat is not the problem. It's the sugary and ultra-processed food in combination with stress that almost put me six feet under." He took his plastic fork and knife and cut a piece of the enormous double burger.

"What do you mean?" she asked.

"There's a lot of new research that too much sugar and starch in your diet causes your pancreas to ramp up insulin production to take the sugar out of your bloodstream and into your cells. Too much will make your cells resistant, and that's why you end up with chronic high blood sugars. This, in turn, causes systemic issues that you see in many diabetics, such as kidney disease, blindness, and huge blood sugar swings. That's why I keep sugar, bread, and starchy foods out of my diet—to take a load off of my pancreas and let my cells recover. That's why I now consider myself a diabetic in remission."

"But what about all the fat," she repeated. "Doesn't that clog your arteries?"

"Again, the fat is not the problem. It's the effect of highly processed, carb-y foods. You see, consuming starches and sugary foods and drinks also increase inflammation in your body. As a result, your arteries get damaged. Cholesterol, what most think is blocking arteries, is actually repairing the damage done…"

"I think you lost me at the pancreas," Jenna said.

"Sorry, I got carried away again. I am much healthier eating the way I do now than I was half a year ago. Trust me, and I have the test results to prove it."

"Okay, I'll take your word, even though I still can't wrap my head around how your dinner can be healthy. I hope you don't mind me eating my burger and those wonderful fries." She cringed as soon as the words left her mouth. "Sorry."

He laughed. "No worries. Even though I miss fries, my burger is very satisfying."

When they finished their meal, Jenna closed the lid of her box. "I'm stuffed, but we have some work to do, or we'll be here all night."

He wouldn't mind that at all, but he thought better of than saying it out loud. Instead, he stood up, grabbed the boxes and cleared off the table.

As Cody unpacked the ingredients for the cupcakes and set them out on the counter, Jenna studied the recipe he had printed out for her and penciled in a few notes. "What do you think?" he asked. If anyone could make this a tasty treat for his patients, and possibly for himself, occasionally, it was her.

Jenna nodded as she finished reading through the directions. "It's a fairly simple recipe, and if we tweak a couple of the ingredients, I think we can lighten the texture and definitely improve on the mouth-feel."

This was going better than he had expected. "Great! Shall we get started then?"

"I'm ready," she said with a smile, "but I'll need you to do most of the work."

"Understood. What's first?" he asked, eager to get started.

"First, let's gather all the ingredients, bowls, and pans we need," she said. "Bowls and muffin pans are down to your left. I'll preheat the oven in the meantime," she said as she walked over to the industrial multi-cavity appliance.

He scratched his head when he saw the many sizes of bowls in front of him, but then opted for a medium bowl for the batter and a small bowl for the icing, close to what he used at home to make his batch. He also grabbed a large and a small muffin pan, just in case.

"Perfect," she said and grabbed a wooden spoon from the utensil container on the counter and some measuring cups. "First, let's start with the dry ingredients."

Cody had to admit, he enjoyed working on their project together. She taught him how to prepare the batter and why certain ingredients work well in baking and why substituting an ingredient can sometimes mean success or epic fail.

"It's all about the physical properties and chemical reactions that make a tasty cupcake," she said as she scooped a tablespoon of baking powder into his batter.

He smiled. "Chemistry. Now you're talking my language." Before tonight, baking was a mystery to him. If he wanted something sweet, which was most afternoons and evenings prior to his heart attack, he had his preferred spots where he could pick up a pie, donuts, or else make a batch of brownies at home. Tonight, Jenna showed him through science how to build a masterpiece. At least, he hoped so.

"Okay, we're almost done with the batter," she said. "I'll prepare the muffin pan, and you can pour the batter into the cups for me."

Cody couldn't help it, but he glanced at her as she lined the muffin pan with colorful paper cups. A strand of her strawberry-blonde hair had escaped from her messy bun and hung loosely down the side of her face. It took all he had to resist tucking that strand of hair behind her ear.

"All right," she said. "Now carefully fill each of the cups two-thirds full with batter."

He closed the distance between them to reach the muffin pan better and noticed she only moved a few inches to the side to give him room. His palpitations returned. *There goes my heart again,* he thought. With slightly shaky hands, he poured the batter into the cups. Small dots of the yellow dough dripped on the side of the pan.

"No worries," Jenna said, wiping them off with a quick swipe of a damp cloth she kept nearby. "We don't want it to bake on the pan and burn."

She glanced up at him, and their eyes met. For a moment, neither one broke the gaze.

The temptation to kiss her was overwhelming. Cody wasn't sure how long he could prevail.

The oven beeped.

Jenna flinched. "It finished preheating," she said, her voice raspy.

Saved by the bell, he thought.

She cleared her throat. "Let's get the cupcakes in the oven, and then we'll start on the icing."

"Right," he said, his voice equally scratchy.

As the cupcakes baked, Cody's concentration was shot. He couldn't believe that he almost kissed her. Just because they finally found some common ground didn't mean that he should allow his feelings to go rampant and risk a potential partnership with her that could give his metabolically impaired patients a tasty alternative to the potentially lethal options. No, he had to remain professional for the town's sake.

"What color of icing and flavor do you prefer?" she asked him after the basic icing was ready.

"I'm the wrong person to ask." He thought for a moment. "We should approach this logically. For your diabetic customers, which cupcake is the bestselling one?"

She thought for a moment. "The lemon cheesecake cupcakes sell very well among my older customers. They like the more traditional varieties."

"Why don't we start there, then?" he suggested.

Jenna walked to the fridge and retrieved a pack of cream cheese. "If we do the regular recipe of icing and substitute the sugar with your sweetener and adjust the amount, we should be able to replicate the recipe fairly easy."

"Let's try it." He reached for the smaller bowl.

"No, let's use the mixer for this. You'll thank me later," she said.

Once the icing formed beautiful peaks, Jenna stopped the mixer and pulled the bowl out from under the beaters.

The oven timer beeped again.

"Can you pull out the cupcakes for me?" Jenna asked. "The mitts are next to the oven."

Cody opened the oven door, and the wonderful aroma of freshly baked cupcakes enveloped him. He took another whiff, then pulled out the tray of perfect mounds of golden cupcakes.

"Just set them on the counter for a minute, and then we'll let them cool on a wire rack," she instructed. "Once they have cooled, we can decorate them with the icing. If they are still warm, the icing will melt, and we'll wind up with a hot mess."

Cody did as she told him. He couldn't wait to taste the

finish product, and he couldn't wait to see if Jenna liked them. If she would give her approval, he was certain that his patients would like them, too. After all, she knew her customers better than he did.

"I have an idea," Jenna said. "Why don't we melt some baking chocolate, add a dash of vanilla, and add some of your sweetener to make sugar-free decorations we can stick into the icing?"

Cody's corners of his lips turned up into a smile. "I like the way you think. You can never go wrong with chocolate."

Jenna grabbed a small glass bowl and broke off a few squares of baking chocolate and microwaved it for a few seconds to melt it. She then added the remaining ingredients. Next, she tore off a square of parchment paper and lined a baking sheet with it. Finally, she slowly poured a thin stream of the chocolate mixture, using her good arm, to create a swirly pattern on the parchment that to Cody resembled an artful sketch of a ball of yarn. "Let's store the chocolate decorations in the fridge for now," she said, "so they can firm up."

Cody carried the baking sheet to the fridge. "How long will they have to stay in there?" he asked.

"Just a few minutes," she said.

Once the decorations cooled and hardened, Jenna picked one up and broke it in half. "Here, try it," she said, handing Cody a small piece.

He turned it in his hand to inspect it from all sides. "It looks delicate and delicious," he said, then popped it in his mouth, where it slowly melted. "Oh, this is so good."

Jenna did the same with hers. "Yes, it is. It's just the right mix."

Their gazes met again, and Cody noticed a stirring in his chest, similar to when he was waiting for his medical board results. His first instinct was to grab one of Jenna's cupcakes, but he knew that food wouldn't cure his insecurities, although it was tempting to ease his discomfort.

Jenna broke their gaze, straightened her apron, and checked the cupcakes that had been cooling on the cooling rack. "Uhm, I think we can start decorating them," she said. "I can't hold my arm up that high yet, so you'll have to do it for me."

"I can't guarantee that they'll look anything like yours when they're done," he said. "Remember the ones I brought in?"

Jenna giggled. "Sorry, but yes, I do. Don't worry, though, these are prototypes and just for us."

"I'll do my best." Cody took the filled icing bag and followed Jenna's instructions. At first a large blob of icing shot from the tip of the bag. "Argh!"

"Easy, cowboy!" she said. "A little lighter on the squeezing action will do the trick. You'll get the hang of it."

He tried again, and this time, the flow of the icing was more fluid. Cody hovered the bag in a circular motion over the cupcake as he tried to evenly distribute the icing. Unfortunately, his circles were uneven, and a few strands were hanging over the edge of the cupcakes like garlands. "I'm not good at this," he said when he was about to admit defeat.

"Nonsense," she replied. "It just takes practice." With her good hand, she gently guided his, and the circles became more uniform.

He was highly aware of her hand touching his arm.

Come on, Cody. Focus on the cupcakes, he thought. Easier said than done.

When they finished, they stepped back to admire their work. Jenna grabbed the chocolate balls of yarn, as he called them, and together they topped each cupcake with the chocolate to give them the finishing touch.

"These are perfect for Ms. Maggie's craft shop," he said.

"I agree. They turned out beautiful. And not too shabby for a newbie cupcake baker," she teased him. "Let's try them."

They each took one cupcake off the cooling rack.

Cody turned his to admire it from all sides, peeled off the paper, then took a bite. To his surprise, the consistency was much lighter than of those he had baked the other day. Also, the icing was light and delicious and had just the right amount of sweetness. It wasn't overpowering at all. "These are awesome," he said with his mouth full. "No wonder my patients can't resist."

She smiled. "Remember, it's all about getting the chemistry right."

Cody noticed a dab of icing stuck to her lip. "Wait, you've got something there." He raised his thumb to her mouth and wiped away the extra icing. Not sure where to put it, he licked it off his thumb, unable to take his gaze off her eyes. When she closed them and leaned forward, all his earlier intentions of keeping this relationship purely professional evaporated, and he met her halfway until their lips touched.

"Jenna, are you okay?" a voice approached from the front of the shop.

They sprang apart.

"Oh, hi Sean," she said, pulling a strand of hair out of her face.

Sean assessed the situation. "Oh, Cody. I was just making sure everything is okay. Jenna rarely stays this late."

Jenna straightened her apron. "I'm all right."

Sean cleared this throat. "Well, since everything seems to be in order, I'll be on my way." He tipped his hat. "Jenna, Cody, glad you're okay. I will see you around."

As soon as the sheriff left, they broke out into laughter. "We better clean up here."

CHAPTER TWELVE

*E*arly Monday morning, a well-rested Jenna unlocked the door of her bakery. Clarissa drove up around the same time Jenna went back to her car to grab a cupcake container. If today went well, she would walk over to Cody's practice to let him know about her decision to offer the new line of cupcakes in her shop. Her shoulder had healed even more over the weekend, and her range of motion without pain improved every day.

"Mornin', Jenna. Whatcha got there?" Clarissa asked, without her usual perky and borderline annoying voice as she held the door for her.

As Jenna passed, Clarissa sneaked a peek through the opaque colored lid of the carrier.

"A surprise," Jenna teased. "I'll let you all try when Willow and Beth get here."

"Is it a new flavor of cupcakes?" Clarissa asked.

"Just wait and see. You'll get to try it." Jenna set the container down on the counter, then turned to Clarissa. "Are you okay? You look exhausted."

"I'm fine, my dear," Clarissa replied. "I'll get started on today's cupcakes in a minute," she added with a long yawn.

Her unusual demeanor worried her. "Did you not sleep well?"

"To be honest, I'm exhausted. I've been baking pies all weekend to make some extra money to pay our bills, and getting up early, too, on top of my regular job is wearing on me."

As much as Jenna didn't like Clarissa early on, as she got to know her, she almost felt sorry for her. She tried to hold it all together—her appearances, her social status, and their finances. "I really appreciate you coming in to decorate for me in the mornings. We probably would've had to shut down without your help while I'm healing."

"It's fine. I really need the money right now."

Jenna thought for a moment. "I have an idea. Everyone in town raves about your cakes and pies. Give me a week until I can do all my own baking again, and we can work out a deal. You could bake your cakes and pastries at home and on your off-time, and I can sell them here at the shop on consignment. We've been running short on inventory, and a consignment model would work well for both of us. What do you say?"

"That would be wonderful," Clarissa said with a weary smile. "I just feel like I'm burning my candles on both ends to pay the bills right now."

Jenna could relate. The hours she had been putting into her bakery since she made her dream a reality were innumerable. How many times had she barely made it home after almost falling asleep at the wheel? "I get it, Clarissa."

The chime of the front door rang. "Good morning,"

Beth called out and walked into the kitchen, followed by Willow, whose hair was a bright purple today. "Oh, what's this?" she asked, pointing at Jenna's cupcake container.

Jenna smiled. "A surprise. But now that you're all here…" She unlatched the sides of the container and lifted the lid. "This is the prototype of the doctor-approved lemon cheesecake cupcakes. I made a fresh batch last night."

"Those look yummy," Willow said. "Are those for us? I'm just asking, because I didn't eat breakfast yet."

"It's not exactly a breakfast food," Beth added, "but I'll give 'em a try. May I?" she asked.

"Of course. Go for it," Jenna said and waited for their reaction with bated breath.

"Doctor-approved, huh?" Clarissa said. "Are they low fat?"

Jenna shook her head. "No, they are actually low carb for Dr. Walker's diabetes patients. They are sugar free, and we used almond flour instead of regular flour."

Clarissa sneered. "How is that supposed to be good?"

"Don't knock it before you try it," Willow said, taking a bite herself.

Beth licked the icing off her lips. "Not half bad," she said.

"Thank you," Jenna said. "It's not quite the same texture as our regular cupcakes, but it's a very close match to the original version."

Clarissa took a bite of her cupcake, and Jenna watched her facial expression relax. "Better than I expected, actually."

Jenna let out her breath. If Clarissa, with her refined taste, liked them, she knew they were onto something.

"You should make an entire line of them," Willow suggested. "We could make a sign: *Made with Love and Doctor-Approved* with a picture of a heart and a stethoscope. You know, like a logo."

"I like the sound of that." Jenna replied. "We might have to keep you working here as long as we can. You're creative and have come up with so many great ideas so far."

"Yep, she's a keeper," Beth chimed in.

"Let's put them in the display shelf and see if they sell. Willow, do you want to make the sign?"

Willow smiled. "Of course. We should also cut up one or two cupcakes and offer samples."

"Great idea," Jenna said.

When Willow and Clarissa got busy with their work, Beth pulled Jenna aside and whispered so the others couldn't hear. "So, are those the cupcakes you made on your baking date with Cody?"

Jenna's face warmed. "It wasn't a date, even though he brought dinner. It was like a business meeting, and we fine-tuned a recipe. That's all."

"Not what I hear from Sean," Beth said, wagging her finger.

Jenna made a mental note to strangle him next time she saw him—sheriff or not. "Sean knows nothing," she hissed back at her friend.

"Why are you getting so upset? Since the tornado, you've been unusually chipper, considering the circumstances, and I bet the new doc has something to do with that," Beth mused. "For enemies, you two get along quite well, but that's me just thinking out loud."

"Well, you can stop thinking, Beth. There's nothing going on between us."

"Whatever you say," Beth said. "I'm going to help Clarissa with the cupcakes for today."

Jenna closed her eyes, trying to remember the moment Cody had almost kissed her Friday evening just before Sean busted in on them. His timing had been horrible, and neither Jenna nor Cody had mentioned it after Sean left. Instead, the rest of their bake-date, as Beth called it, ended awkwardly, to say the least.

Her phone buzzed in her back pocket.

"Hello, Ms. Wilson. This is Trey from Kendricks Construction," the male voice on the other end of the line said. "Ma'am, I just wanted to call and let you know that we're at your house and are starting the repair job on your roof and wall. If the weather holds up, we should finish by Wednesday or Thursday."

"Thank you for the update," Jenna replied. "I assume you found the key?"

"Yes, ma'am. I have a couple of my guys work inside. We will clean up after ourselves tonight before we leave," the man said. "I will also keep you updated throughout the day if any issues come up."

"Thank you," she said. She ended the call and joined Clarissa and Beth in the kitchen to bake a few more batches of cupcakes for the day.

By mid-morning, Jenna saw Maggie entering the store. "Hello, young lady," she said to Willow. "Weren't you in our knitting class the other evening?"

"Yes, ma'am. I almost finished my scarf."

"That's wonderful," Maggie replied, her voice much

more cheerful now. "You should bring it next time and show it off."

"I will, Ms. Maggie."

Jenna watched as Willow pointed at the cupcake samples. Despite her first hesitation to hire the young woman with the colorful hair and black combat boots, she knew she had found a gem.

"Would you like to try a sample of our new line of Doctor-Approved cupcakes?" Willow continued. "This is a low-carb version of our customer favorite—the lemon cheesecake cupcake. The recipe is inspired and approved by Dr. Walker himself and is meant to offer an alternative for his diabetic patients and anyone who wants a healthier version of our original cupcakes."

By now, both Beth and Jenna poked their heads out of the kitchen as Maggie took a sample.

Maggie stuck her toothpick in the cake part and put it in her mouth. "Hm. This is delicious. And you said Doc Walker approved this?"

"Yes, ma'am. He did," Willow replied.

"If that's so, I'd like to take two of them—one for myself and one for my daughter, Anna. Also, add one of those birthday cake cupcakes for my granddaughter. Maybe next time we have a knitting session at the shop, I'll buy a couple of the Doctor-Approved ones in addition to the regular cupcakes for the ladies."

Willow packed Maggie's cupcakes in a box and took her payment.

As soon as Maggie left, Beth and Jenna stormed out of the kitchen and high-fived Willow.

"I didn't know you had that much selling talent, Willow," Beth said.

Jenna grinned from ear to ear. "I couldn't have done it any better. Great job! I feel so blessed to have you join us. You have so many hidden talents, and I can't wait to see what wonderful surprises come next."

Willow looked down to the floor. "Thank you, Miss Wilson."

"It's Jenna, remember?"

"Yes, ma'am."

"Keep up the excellent work!" Jenna said and clapped her hands on her thighs. "All right, ladies, let's get back to work. We've got to bake a few more batches for Clarissa to decorate in the morning."

Later that afternoon, only Beth and Jenna remained in the shop preparing for the next day. Willow had left about an hour ago to see her college advisor in Savannah about her next term.

"Hey, Jenna, look at this," Beth called from the shop door.

Jenna came out of the kitchen and joined Beth. "What's up?"

Beth pointed to Cody's car across the street. Cody came out first, then opened the passenger door for a pretty, slender woman with long light brown hair. She looked as if she was in her late twenties. They walked toward the clinic laughing. His hand lay on her back as he guided her through the door to his practice. The door shut behind them, and they disappeared.

Jenna's chest tightened with that familiar sensation of shame. How could she have been so gullible to slowly fall for him? He was a player, and she should've known better. Her spidey senses had tried to warn her, but she had ignored them. Thank goodness they only barely kissed

Friday night. "I told you so, Beth," she said to her friend and walked back into the kitchen. "Come on, we've got some more work to do before it's time to go home."

So much for heading over to tell Cody that she was going to offer the low-carb cupcakes for his patients, she thought. She glanced at her empty container she had carried the cupcakes in this morning. Images of the baking-date and their almost-kiss flashed through her mind. How foolish she had been—foolish enough to have him talk her into a new line of cupcakes, which translated into more work and expensive ingredients. Neither one she could afford. Maybe it was a bad idea altogether to offer the low-carb line.

~

*A*s every Monday, Cody had been busy most of the day taking care of walk-in patients. The weather was cooling off now, and he saw more sniffles and coughs than he had his entire time in Magnolia Hill, which hadn't been long. But today he was determined to carve out some time to head over to Jenna's shop to talk more about the trial run of their low-carb cupcakes.

He was surprised, though, that he didn't hear from her one way or another over the weekend, especially after their near kiss on Friday evening. Granted, there was still an awkward cloud looming above and between them. Maybe she was busy with the repair of her house.

Then he realized that this went both ways. He had spent most of the weekend installing another obstacle in his backyard. What he should've done was take the time to call and check on her or even drive by her house to see if she needed help with anything. To be honest, he didn't know what he should do. Cody had been out of the dating game since college, except for a few attempts in his residency. But working long shifts and odd hours at the clinic weren't quite compatible with finding someone who, like him, was in it for the long-haul. He was raised traditional and was looking for a soulmate. With his work schedule, it seemed impossible. Now that he finally had the time to date, he didn't know where to start. He didn't want to be too forward with Jenna and risk her getting mad at him again.

He checked his watch. It was already three o'clock. Where did the time go? "When's my next appointment?" he asked Twyla as he refilled his tumbler at the water cooler in the waiting room.

Twyla wiggled the mouse to wake the computer. "In about twenty minutes, Dr. Walker," she said. "Did you know there is a buzz going around town about a new *doctor-approved cupcake?*" she asked with a telling smile, giving away that she knew something.

Playing along, he put on his rusty southern charm. "Is that so, Ms. Twyla?"

"Yes, sir," she said, emphasizing the sir. "And I'm gonna try me one before I go home today."

"Then you might want to hurry over and buy enough for our staff before they sell out," he said, handing her a twenty. "It's on me." This would've been his chance to talk to Jenna, but he wanted to wait until later in the afternoon when they both were less busy.

"Thanks, doctor," she said. She rushed out the door and almost ran poor Mrs. Riley over. "I'm so sorry," she said to the elderly woman. "I was just going across the street for an afternoon snack. Let's go in and get you checked in."

"Hello, Mrs. Riley," Cody greeted her. "Twyla, it's okay, I'll take care of her." He shooed his receptionist away. He walked around the desk and clicked on a few buttons on Twyla's computer screen, but soon realized that he was out of his league.

Press yes to delete records, the small window on her screen prompted.

He'd better leave it alone before he accidentally deleted his entire patient database. Twyla would never forgive him. "Come on, Mrs. Riley." He grabbed the woman's record off Twyla's desk. "Let's get you into a room."

"Thank you, Doctor. I'm sorry; I came in early."

"That's no problem at all," he said. "Let's get your weight, blood pressure, and see how you're doing."

After the appointment, Cody walked Mrs. Riley to the front. "Twyla will fix everything I messed up in her computer and will set up your next appointment."

Twyla shot him a glare, then rolled her eyes at him as she clicked and typed away on her keyboard. "Mrs. Riley, we already have you scheduled for next Monday at two p.m.—same as today."

"Thank you, Miss Twyla," the old woman said. "Say hello to your momma from me."

"I certainly will," she said.

"Goodbye, Dr. Walker." Mrs. Riley poked her head over the colorful box on the receptionist's desk. "Oh, this looks like my favorite cupcake, except it has a beautiful dainty chocolate decor on it and a little sign on a toothpick. I'm afraid I can't read it with my tired old eyes."

"The sign says *Made with Love and Doctor-Approved*," Twyla said.

The woman's face lit. "Oh, are those the new cupcakes Dr. Walker wants us to eat that the entire town is talking about?"

"They are, Mrs. Riley," Cody said. "But they are meant as an occasional special treat and not to eat three a day."

The old woman clutched her purse. "I will visit Miss Jenna across the street and take some home for myself and my Frank."

"You better hurry," Twyla said. "There were only two left."

Both smiled as Mrs. Riley waved at them and hurried across the street to the Cherry on Top bakery.

"Looks like the new cupcakes are a hit," Twyla said and opened the lid of the box.

Cody was amazed how artfully the icing swirled to a peak. The chocolate ball of yarn he made Friday evening looked nothing like this delicate chocolate design that adorned the top of the cream-color icing. The sign Mrs. Riley had referred to was an elegantly shaped card stock tag with a blue border, depicting a red heart and a stethoscope.

"What a genius idea," Twyla said as she pulled a cupcake out of the box and pulled the little sign out. "Girls, come get you a treat!" she called to the rest of the clinic staff.

The more Cody witnessed the excitement about the new treats, the more certain he was that his business relationship between him and Jenna would be a success. Maybe they could expand the flavors and not just limit the healthy option to just one kind. He couldn't wait until his last patient would arrive, because that meant that he would finally have time to run over to see Jenna after work and tell her about this good news. But first he was going to indulge in a treat.

"These are so good!" Cindy, his lab tech, said.

Cody took the last cupcake left in the box. He couldn't wait to try it. First, he peeled off the colorful dotted paper off the sides and bottom, then took his first bite. As soon as the icing and the fluffy cake hit his mouth, he was in heaven. Whatever Jenna did to improve on Friday's recipe worked. Cody could taste extra lemon flavor in the bready part of the treat, and the creamy cheesecake icing complemented the flavors perfectly. That woman had a gift. And now, he could indulge in something sweet every once in a while, without risking landing on a stretcher in the ER again, unless he injured himself in his outdoor backyard ninja gym.

The office phone rang, and Twyla answered. "Dr. Walker's practice."

Cody polished off his cupcake and licked his lips. He didn't feel the sugar-rush he would get from a regular donut. Instead, his stomach was comfortably full, and his craving for sweets was satisfied.

"Dr. Walker," Twyla said. "Your last appointment, Mr. Smith, had to reschedule."

Excellent. This meant he could see Jenna now. Cody loved it when everything fell into place. "On that note, ladies, why don't you wrap up what you're doing and call it an early afternoon. Unless something earth-shattering is happening in the next hour, we're good to go."

He didn't have to wait long before all of his employees had gone home. Cody hung his lab coat on the rack and put on a light jacket. On his way out, he locked the door to his practice. With a swing in his step, he was about to head over to see Jenna when Mrs. Wallace stopped him on the sidewalk. He noticed she had a slight limp when she walked.

"Hello Dr. Walker," the old woman said, and started talking about days gone by when she was a teacher and watching everyone local to Magnolia Hill grow up.

He resisted checking his watch, and he didn't have the heart to walk away from the ninety-year-old sweet lady.

"You know, Doctor, I've been having this knee pain lately I need to get looked at. I think I twisted it this morning when I was sweeping my front porch."

Cody glanced across the street. What he wanted to do was talk to Jenna, but he couldn't just turn Mrs. Wallace away and tell her to make an appointment tomorrow. "You're already here. Why don't I have a quick look at your knee right now?"

"Oh, Dr. Walker, you don't have to go out of your way…" she said.

Cody smiled. "No worries. I just want to make sure you're okay." Too many times he'd seen elderly patients underplay their injuries. "It'll only take a few minutes." Cody unlocked the door to his practice and invited her in.

"If you insist," she said.

Thirty minutes later, Mrs. Wallace left his practice with a smile. "Thank you, Dr. Walker, for taking a look. I will see you at my next appointment," she said and left.

Cody locked up the behind him again. He glanced across the street, but this time, Jenna's SUV was gone. He walked to her shop and checked the front door, but it was locked. *Maybe she's still in the kitchen,* he thought.

Cody knocked on the glass, but again, there was no answer.

With his head hung low, he walked to his car. It wasn't that he regretted taking care of Mrs. Wallace; he was looking forward to talking to Jenna all afternoon, and now he had missed his chance.

CHAPTER THIRTEEN

While Beth and Willow went to Mamaw's to pick up lunch, Jenna ordered several more bags of almond flour and monk fruit sweetener in bulk from her main supplier. She had thought long and hard last night if she should continue offering the new line of cupcakes. It only made good business sense, as fast as they had flown off the shelves, so Beth helped her whip up another double batch. Willow's idea with the toothpick signs also paid off.

Even though she was excited about the sudden success, she also had doubts. Every batch she made reminded her of the evening with Cody. It also reminded her how he had escorted that sorority chick into his practice. She couldn't trust him as far as she could throw him.

Jenna didn't know why she was so upset. Technically, they didn't really kiss. It wasn't like they were officially dating, either. Every day she met Cody was like a roller coaster. First, he busted into her shop and accused her of killing his patients, then he was all nice about rescuing her from the tornado. *Well, it is his job after all*; she thought. Checking on her in the ER and letting her stay in his guest room wasn't. She smashed the ball of pie dough on the counter with her good arm. By now she figured out what she could get away with her injured shoulder, and she reserved dough smashing for her good arm.

The front door chimed, and Beth and Willow walked in, looking somewhat uncomfortable.

"What's going on? Long line at Mamaw's?"

Beth nudged Willow with her elbow. "You tell her."

"Uh, no," Willow replied. "You tell her. She's your friend, remember?"

"Tell me what?" Jenna said, sensing she wouldn't like a bit what they were about to tell her.

Beth took a deep breath. "Cody was at the diner when we got there."

"So? Even he has to eat sometimes. There's nothing unusual about that," Jenna said.

Beth shifted from one leg to the other. "He was there with the same woman that came to his practice after hours earlier this week."

"Oh?" This only confirmed that he wasn't that interested in her, and he was just using her for the cupcakes. "He can have lunch with whoever he wants. We just have a common business goal—cupcakes."

"But I thought you and him…" Beth whispered.

Jenna laughed. Maybe it sounded too over-the-top to make it believable. "There was nothing going on between us," she said, hoping her mind would believe it if she spoke the words often enough. "Go ahead and eat your lunch. I need to finish this pie."

The women took their takeout boxes to the table in the

back of the kitchen and ate their food in silence while Jenna lined a pie form with the dough.

She must've been in a zone the last few hours, because before she knew it, Willow had left at the end of her shift, and Beth joined her in the kitchen.

"Look, I'm sorry for being such a downer," Jenna said. "I just don't know where I stand with Cody. For a moment I thought we were heading in the right direction, and now I'm kicking myself for being so gullible."

The door chimed again and, with some clanking and popping, Kevin entered the bakery with a hand truck stacked with boxes. "Hello ladies, I have your deliveries," he said as he rolled the load of boxes into the kitchen. As he passed Beth, he stole a quick kiss from her and winked at Jenna. He was a welcomed fresh breath of air every time he dropped off her orders.

Beth had found a good man, one that cared about her deeply, Jenna thought. One who was good-natured, and his clumsiness was downright charming. She longed for a kind of relationship they shared. It just wasn't her time yet. Would it ever be?

As soon as he came, Kevin and his empty hand truck left the bakery—but not without stealing another kiss from Beth, asking what's for dinner, and bumping the door on the way out.

Both laughed once he was out of earshot.

"You are so lucky," Jenna said to Beth. "I want someone like your Kevin, but every time I get my hopes up, something happens, and I'm alone again."

Beth gently rubbed her back. "You survived a tornado, Jenna. That's a big deal. Look at all that you've accomplished since then: you've kept the shop open, you almost have that skylight in your bedroom fixed, and you've launched a highly successful cupcake line with lots of potential. So what if Cody is being a jerk? Your true love will come around soon enough."

Jenna tried to smile, although her eyes likely revealed her disappointment. "You know, Beth, once I got to know Cody better, I really thought this could work. You know how I get these vibes about couples. I was right about you and Kevin, and I was right about Anna and Jason. Oddly enough, after the tornado, I thought he was the one. But him meeting in public with this woman, in a small town where rumors fly, this just confirms that my vibes mean nothing when it comes to my own love life. I'll just have to accept that it's not meant to be."

"Speaking of…" Beth said, pointing at the door. "Your not-meant-to-be is here."

A jolt of anxiety coursed through her body. He still looked handsome, she had to give him that, but in light of the recent sightings, she was not interested in playing second fiddle or competing for his favor. If she would enter into a relationship with someone, he only should have eyes for her. Obviously, this wasn't the case with Cody.

"Are you okay?" Beth asked.

"I'm fine," Jenna replied, even though the little angel and the little devil sitting on her shoulders filled her mind with conflicting messages, which resulted in a wild swirl of thoughts.

Beth touched her good shoulder. "Well, this is my cue. I'm heading home so you two can have some privacy to talk. See you tomorrow morning." Beth grabbed her purse and left with a "Hello, Dr. Walker," as she passed him.

"Hi, Jenna," he said with a timid smile. "Can I come into the kitchen?"

"Hello, Cody," she said. "Come on in. I'm just finishing up these pies."

He entered the kitchen and stopped in front of the work surface they had experimented on with his cupcakes last week.

The moment of their almost-kiss flashed through her mind, but she tried to force out that memory. She had to stay strong. His niceness could not get the best of her. She had learned her lesson with him.

"Looks like you're regaining some mobility in your shoulder," he said. "How's the pain?"

"Better, thank you," she said. "What can I help you with?"

"I just wanted to tell you that my patients and my staff are raving about your low-carb cupcakes," he said. "I had one when Twyla picked up a box for the practice, and whatever you did to the recipe, it turned out wonderful."

"Thank you again," she said. "I've added a squirt of lemon extract to the batter and played with the other ingredients some more. I think this will be the final version. My customers seem to like it."

"So, you'll continue making them?" he asked.

Jenna paused to choose her words wisely. She had to do what was right for her business and the town. The cupcakes sold well, her customers loved them, and they didn't mind paying a little extra. She'd have to get over herself and her hurt feelings. "Yes. I will continue the line —for the time being—and possibly offer a variety of flavors if there's demand. We'll see how it goes."

He came around the counter and drew her in a tight bearhug. "Thank you, Jenna! This means the world to me."

Even though she didn't want to, her logical mind took over, and she wiggled her way out of his embrace. Jenna straightened her apron. "Let's keep this professional."

Cody took a step back and blushed. "Sorry. Yes, of course." He looked flustered. "I'm just excited about you helping my patients and me out on this."

"That's what I do. I bake."

~

*A*fter a rigorous Friday morning workout in his backyard, Cody sipped on his coffee. He still didn't know what he'd done wrong that changed Jenna's mind about him. Had he been too forward last week with that attempt at a kiss? He wasn't sure. Maybe he should've followed up with her on the weekend to see if she needed anything—just being neighborly. But he didn't even do that. Instead, he had buried himself in projects around his own house. Cody didn't like stepping outside of his comfort zone, and he was definitely there with Jenna. In the past, feeling out of his element drove him to comfort food. He no longer had that luxury if he wanted to live. And he did. He had to find out what happened and make up for it this weekend, if it was his fault. Maybe he'd stop by her house with yet another peace offering, hoping they could clear out the awkwardness between them.

Cody took a quick shower, made a breakfast roll-up out of deli meat, cheese, a squirt of mayo and a few dots of mustard, and wrapped it all up in a large lettuce leaf. He pickup up the weekly local paper off the driveway and tossed it on the passenger seat of his car. Cody enjoyed reading the paper. As a newcomer in town, he wanted to learn as much as he could about the community and important events. His dad had passed that nugget of wisdom on to him when he entered med school. 'If you know your patients, you can relate better, and in turn, you'll find they trust you more.' This advice had served him well so far. Too bad his dad never took the time away from his work to get to know him better.

He sat in his car and glanced over at the paper. The rubber band that held it together had snapped, and the front-page headline glared at him. *New Doctor at War with Local Cupcake Shop.*

Cody's heart stopped. "What the…?" He snatched the newspaper off the seat and unfolded it to read the article. With each line, his chest tightened, and blood pulsed through his veins like a raging wild river. He pulled his phone out of his pocket, searched for the number of the Magnolia Hill Herald, and dialed the number.

"Magnolia Hill Herald, this is Miriam Sue Webster," the voice said on the other end of the line.

"Why did you print this article?" he yelled into the phone. "I retracted it two weeks ago."

"Ah, Dr. Walker," she said with a smug tone in her voice. "I was wondering how long it would take for you to call."

"That doesn't answer my question. Why did you print it? And that made-up headline was not what this article was about. My article is about helping my patients, the people of your town."

"It was a slow week, and you only left a message on

my answering machine, which somehow got erased, and I simply forgot about it. Plus, it was an excellent piece."

The temperature of Cody's blood reached the boiling point. "That's a lie!" he fumed. "Take it off!"

She laughed. "Well, it's too late now. The article has already printed, and the entire town has received their copy."

"You'll just have to print an apology in the next issue, or I'll sue you. You just ruined my reputation." He'd be lucky if he had any patients left by the time he got to his practice this morning.

"Now, now," Miriam Sue said with a calm voice. "Let's not get ahead of ourselves. You sent me that article to print. I admit, I edited the headline."

"My article was an opinion piece in a small column, not splashed all over the front page. Also, I recalled it."

"Do you have proof of that?"

He didn't. Maybe with call tracing through the phone company he could dig out something, but right now it didn't look good for him. For now, all he could do was bite the bullet and chalk it up to poor judgement on his end. Lesson learned—a tough lesson at that. "Issue a public and sincere apology in next week's paper and I might drop the defamation lawsuit. You know you were wrong for publishing it."

Miriam Sue sighed. "Well, okay, I apologize, and I will write a correction in the next issue." She paused. "Are you still planning on writing a monthly health column? One of my contributors left, and I need to fill her space."

He couldn't believe that she had the nerve to ask him for help after what she had done to him. "You've got to be kidding! We're done here."

Cody almost poked a hole into his cell phone when he hung up on her and tossed it onto the passenger seat. He leaned back into his seat and closed his eyes, trying to digest what had happened in the last fifteen minutes of what had promised to be a decent end of his work week.

The urge to run into his house for food to force the feeling of impending doom out of the pit of his stomach was almost unbearable, yet pointless. His fridge and pantry were full of fresh and healthy foods. There was nothing in his house that he could binge on. Jenna's shop was out of question, and so was any other public place that served comfort or junk food. Besides, unless he wanted to dig his early grave, this wasn't an option, anyway. He had to go to work and face the inevitable fallout of his dumb idea to write that article to begin with. It was going to be ugly, but he couldn't just run away and hide under a rock.

When he arrived at his practice, Twyla's phone was ringing off the hook. She glared at him as if she was going to kill him. He deserved that.

"Let it ring, Twyla. Please gather everyone for a staff meeting in the break room," he said when she was about to answer another call.

She got up from her chair, glared at him, then called out, "The boss wants a meeting."

He'd never seen Twyla mad before, and this didn't bode well.

~

For the first time since the tornado, Jenna was alone in her bakery in the wee hours of the morning. She could do most of her baking again, except for the heavy lifting. When Clarissa was moving around the kitchen like a zombie yesterday morning, she gave her the option to try out the consignment model for her baked goods. The poor woman had been burning her candle on both ends, and she didn't look well. "I'd like to continue from home, if that's okay with you," Clarissa had said. She knew all too well how that felt, and since Willow was a superstar in the front, Beth was a big help with baking in the back.

Around seven thirty, Beth walked in, slamming a paper on the countertop. "Have you read this?" she huffed.

"Read what?" Jenna didn't have time to read the paper, and most times it landed in her trash. She hadn't been a fan of Miriam Sue and couldn't care less what she wrote about. But if Beth got all worked up, something in today's issue must've gone wrong. Maybe Magnolia Hill's Fall Festival got canceled this year. Besides Movies in the Park and the Christmas parade, it was a town favorite. She had a feeling, though, that it was worse than that.

"The article on the front page," she said, pointing her finger at the large, bold headline.

New Doctor at War with Local Cupcake Shop.

"What?" Jenna snatched the paper out from under Beth's finger. Her chest tightened, and her pulse raced as blood rushed through her veins. The article named Dr. Cody Walker as the contributor. Cody. How could he? She knew something was up with him all along. And she knew he would not let up on her. As she skimmed through the article, it was a déjà vu of the day they had met. He accused her of making the people of Magnolia Hills sicker, interfering with his treatment, and how her shop was a major health risk. Jenna's mind was churning with emotions. She was furious, yet tears of betrayal, disappointment, and shame for her own naivete welled up in her eyes. "How could he?" she finally managed.

"I don't know, hun," Beth whispered. "I just don't know."

"I thought we were past this." Jenna wiped her tears, rolled up the paper, then stomped toward the front door. "Hold down the shop for me, will ya?" she said, and with only dignity holding her emotions together, she crossed the street and headed straight into Doc Walker's office.

"Jenna…" Twyla tried to stop her.

"Not now," she snapped as she walked past with her eyes focused straight ahead.

She found Cody leaning back in his office chair, his hands covering his face, then running back over his hair. He shook his head. "This is going to be the end of me," he mumbled.

"It sure is," Jenna said, her arms crossed. It took every ounce of restraint not to strangle him.

Cody jumped out of his skin, then looked at her, stood, and walked toward her. "Look, Jenna, I'm so sorry. This article wasn't supposed to print. I recalled it…"

She didn't want to hear his excuses. "Save it!" Jenna shoved her hands onto her waist. "Is this what you do, riding into town on your high horse from the city, thinking you're better than everybody else in our little town and ruining people's life?" The words that had been on her mind finally came out, raw and unfiltered.

"You're wrong."

"I'm not done yet," she continued. "Do you know what you're doing to my business? If I'm forced to shut down because of your article, you'll put all three of us out of work. Is that what you want? You're taking away a few of the simple pleasures some of us enjoy. Diabetes or not, the people of Magnolia Hill should have a choice of what they want to eat. Just because you came here to save the world doesn't mean we want to be saved. Have you considered that, huh?" The words just kept coming, and she didn't plan on holding back.

"Oh, and I should've known that giving you a chance would be a mistake. How naïve of me." She smacked her forehead to drive home the point.

He held his hands out in front of him at an attempt to calm her, but she wasn't having any of that.

"I was willing to work with you by offering a new line of cupcakes, and this is how you thank me? I thought we were a team. Oh, and remember when you almost kissed me? Was that to sucker me into your scheme, to keep me on your good side?" She shook her head. "I almost believed you cared for me, but then I heard nothing for days from you. Did you delete my number? Did you forget where I live? If you cared, why did you not check and see how the house was coming along or if I need anything? This is how we do things in Magnolia Hill. Also, we do not lead each other on and then woe pretty girls behind your back."

He looked at her with his eyes squinting, as if he was confused. "What?"

She didn't let that shake her. "You know what I'm talking about. Your date you brought into the clinic. And Beth saw you having lunch with her. For being…"

"Stop, Jenna!" he interrupted her, his voice stern. "The article was a mistake. It should've never been printed. And the woman…"

Jenna held out her hand to stop him. "We're done here. Don't talk to me. Don't come to the shop. Stay out of my life, even better, go back to where you came from." She turned and marched out of his practice, ignoring Twyla, who stood in disbelief behind her desk. She had to go, because she was afraid that if she'd let him talk, his explanation would weaken her resolve.

CHAPTER FOURTEEN

*a*fter clinic hours were over, Cody drove home with the goal of throwing himself at a workout that would leave him exhausted enough to make him forget today even existed. How he was going to pull himself out of this mess, he didn't know. At least he had the weekend to figure it out.

On his way home, he passed Jenna's house. He winced at the stab of guilt that pierced his gut. Any hope of him ever getting close to her had evaporated in one blow after another. He really had messed things up this time, considering their history.

Cody noticed that the construction material in Jenna's yard was gone now. At least she had her bedroom back, and he truly was glad for her. Thinking back to what she had said during their encounter at the practice, she had a point. He knew he had gone overboard early on when he had burst into her bakery. It had been his addiction talking, and now that the shoe was on the other foot, he knew exactly how it felt to be accused of something without getting a chance to explain yourself.

Images of a box of donuts and a tub of ice cream invaded his mind. *Tempting,* he thought, but even with a day like today, he could not give in. One single bite of a fresh glazed donut would unleash what he called his monster. He heard somewhere that one bite would be too many and one thousand bites would never be enough. This was certainly true for him. He had survived a heart attack once, and his diabetes was in remission. If he went down the road of eating to suppress his discomfort, he knew he would not be so lucky next time.

Cody pulled up in his driveway and got out of his car. The chill of the early November Georgia breeze made his skin grow goosebumps. *Perfect weather for a high-intensity workout,* he thought. He unlocked his front door, put on his workout clothes, filled his water bottle, and went out the backdoor to his ninja playground. He stretched his muscles and shook his limbs to loosen up, then began running his obstacle course.

After his first round of tire flips, hanging bars, and the climbing wall, he was winded, but it wasn't enough. His emotions were still raw. He'd have enough time for one more round before it would get too dark to see without risking injury, so Cody drank a sip of water, then took another lap around the course.

At the last obstacle, his arms burned, and his legs were about to give out when he noticed a car pull up in his front yard. He watched Sean get out of the vehicle in his uniform. *Great. What now?*

Sean headed over his way. A sense of doom washed

over him. Could his day get any worse? "Hello, Sheriff," he said.

"It's Sean, remember?" the sheriff responded. "I heard you had a rough go of things lately."

"That you can say," Cody said, pulling the bottom of his shirt to his face to dry the sweat. "How can I help you?" Not that he wanted to hear any more bad news.

"Actually, I just got off work and stopped by to see how you were doing. Besides, I wanted to come by and admire the progress of your ninja set-up. I figured today would be a good day to do both—thought you could use someone to talk to."

Relieved, he took another swig of water. "It's getting dark, and I didn't rig any lights yet, but I can show you around tomorrow. I have another obstacle kit delivery scheduled for the morning and could use some help to set it up."

"Count me in," Sean said.

Cody looked down and nodded at Sean's foot. "How is your wound? Any better?"

Sean shifted his weight on his injured foot and bounced on it. "Still sore, but it's healing well." Sean paused, then changed the subject. "So, about the article…"

"I was trying to forget today even existed, but that won't make this situation any better, would it?" Cody said.

Sean wrinkled his forehead. "I'm afraid you might be right."

"Can I offer you something to drink? Water, unsweetened tea, coffee? I'm afraid that's all I have in the house."

"Water will be fine."

They walked through the double sliding doors, and

Sean took a seat at the kitchen table. Cody filled two fresh glasses with ice cubes and cool water from his fridge's water dispenser, then joined Sean at the table.

"So I heard what happened today," Sean began. "Twyla also told me that Miriam Sue gave you a raw deal."

Just that name alone made Cody cringe. When Sean didn't say more, he knew he was waiting for him to talk. As it stood right now, Sean was the only person in town who might care what he had to say. He was his only ally, or as close to one as he could get. Maybe it was a mistake to trust him, but he had no one else to confide in, except for his friend Scott, who never had any downtime working in the ER.

"I had a life-altering medical experience a little over six months ago," Cody began. "You could say that I was clinically dead for a few minutes until they brought me back. A good friend of mine, who worked in the ER when the paramedics brought me in, made it clear that I needed to change my life or the next time I wouldn't be so lucky. I knew that, but I had to hear it from someone else before it sunk in."

"I'm sorry to hear that," Sean said.

"Well, I'm still here, so I did something right," Cody said, attempting a weak smile. "My friend also reminded me how I used to be passionate about sports and saving my patients. Years of stress, long hours, and a long commute each day let me forget what had been important to me as a young physician. I wanted to be a role model for my patients, get to know them, and help them overcome, or at least manage, their diseases. Toward the end of my time in Atlanta, I was so overworked that, I have to admit, I became your typical doctor on autopilot, prescribing medications as Band-Aids. I didn't have the privilege of time to spend with my patients to get to know them better. So, one of my major life changes was to come back to Savannah, where luck had it, Doc Porter was looking for someone to take over his practice."

"So, what happened that got you and Jenna start off on the wrong foot?" Sean asked.

Cody leaned back in his chair. "It was my fault. I was a dummy. After six months of working hard to kick my addiction to food, living a healthy lifestyle, and then coming here, I thought I could get back to my old goals. I got a chance for a do-over, and I would not fail my patients again." He laughed, then shook his head. "Can you believe this food addict sitting in front of you works across the street from a bakery? What's worse, my diabetic patients, the ones I wanted to save from the same fate I barely escaped, had a regular habit of walking straight over to the bakery after they swore off sugar. To me, it felt like a kick in the gut, as if all the cards were stacked against me."

"And your number one problem was Jenna," Sean added. "It makes sense."

"I should've never have let my emotions get the better of me," Cody said. "Instead of being such a knucklehead with blinders on, I should've used my head to come up with a better solution."

"Like the low-carb cupcakes…"

"Yep." Cody shook his head again. "Instead, I waltzed into Jenna's shop like an irrational lunatic threatening to shut her down, worked the Chamber and the BBB to file a complaint—without success, mind you. As a last resort, I wrote the article. I had to, if I wanted to give my patients a chance to reverse their diabetes and improve their quality of life. When Jenna and I worked things out, I immediately called the paper to pull back my article. My bad for not following up on my voicemail with a letter or an email."

"So Miriam Sue printed it anyway?" Sean asked.

"That she did, and then some. She made up a salacious headline. I told her she'd better write an apology and make things right. Can you believe she even asked me to continue writing for her because she's suddenly short on contributors?"

"I can believe it, Cody." Sean took a gulp of his water. "You know, a whole lot of people might be mad at you right now in this town, but give them time. Show them who you really are. I have a hard time believing that you're that jerk everybody believes you are. You'll just have to prove yourself and regain the peoples' trust. Jenna is a very good friend of mine, and I'm here because I saw that sparkle in her eyes. I'm also here because I don't believe for a minute that you're normally that way. Plus," Sean grinned, "I want to work out on your playground."

"Thanks, Sean," Cody said, grateful for his willingness to give him another chance. "Come by tomorrow and we can do a workout. Maybe I can pick your brain of what I need to do legally to cover myself if others want to use my equipment."

"Definitely. I also know an excellent lawyer who can give you some legal advice. Do you mind if I ask Jason to tag along tomorrow?"

Cody laughed. "By all means, if he doesn't hate me, too."

～

*E*xhausted from her crazy day, Jenna fell onto her couch. It was the first opportunity for her to rest and process today's events. What in the world had happened? Why, since this new doctor came to town, did her life get so uprooted in such a short time? Everything was fine before he had arrived. Her business was growing —so much even that she had to hire help. Now, she knew he was serious about shutting her down. Her worst nightmare had become a reality, and she didn't know if she'd still had a bakery a month from now.

At least her customers promised they'd support her. They wouldn't let an outsider harm one of their own, doctor or not. "I will defend you and your shop to my death," Mrs. Riley had promised her when she got her weekly order of cupcakes for herself and her Frank. "Who does this new city doctor think he is, driving into this town and causing a ruckus?" Other customers told her they refuse to have someone tell them they can't have a treat anymore, even though the healthier version was a tasty alternative.

Jenna was grateful for her community's support.

Her phone buzzed in her back pocket. She pulled it out and checked the display before answering. It was Anna. "Hey," she said, deflated.

"Hi, Jenna. How are you feeling?"

"Okay, considering how today went," Jenna replied.

There was a brief pause, then Anna continued. "I worry about you. I don't understand how he could do this to you. You are the least threatening human being in town. You couldn't hurt a fly, even if you tried."

"I know. It's not fair." Jenna sighed. "I just don't know what I can do. I feel so helpless."

"Maybe you need to get a lawyer," Anna suggested. "At least get a consultation."

"I don't know if I can afford one," Jenna said, holding her hand to her forehead. When was this nightmare going to end? "But if things escalate, I might have to find a way."

"Old Mr. Haynes said he'll chase Doc Walker out of town." Anna laughed. "Can you imagine this ninety-five-year-old man running after him with his cane high up in the air?"

Jenna let out a small chuckle when she visualized the scene. "For all I care, he should go right ahead." But deep inside, she knew it was a lie. Even though she was mad as all get out at Cody, it wasn't her nature to wish bad things upon people, no matter how much she despised them.

"Look," Anna said. "I'm off tomorrow. Why don't we have a girls' night out and blow off some steam? We could start with some fine bar food at the Sappy Pine, then break out a deck of cards, and order some wine as I beat your and Beth's butts in rummy. It's been years since we've done that."

Jenna had to agree. She needed to get out and let her hair down. "Okay, I'll go." She paused. "But you forgot, I'm the queen of rummy, not you."

"We shall see, then," Anna teased her. "See you tomorrow evening," she said as they ended the call.

The idea of an evening out lightened her mood. Not that the Sappy Pine was the classiest place in town, but it was a great hangout to spend the evening at and catch up with friends. Anna's invitation gave her something to look forward to—something that would distract her from the horrible events of the last few weeks. She had to admit they weren't all that bad, except for the couple of threats of losing her business over Cody's unreasonable assumption that she was out to kill the residents of Magnolia Hill. And there was that storm. Because of the tornado, she saw a gentle and caring side of Cody. Too bad his actions in the last few days undid all the good that had almost changed her mind about him. *It was for the best,* she told herself.

Jenna stood and walked into the kitchen to pour a glass of tea. She shuddered and almost made a mess when she remembered standing in Cody's office letting him have a piece of her mind. He'd deserved it. But it wasn't like her to fly off the handle like that. She cringed. How could she let herself go like that? Worst of all, she didn't even give him a chance to defend himself. On the other hand, he didn't give her the same courtesy the day he had barged into her shop. Did that make her just as bad of a person? How could she blame him if she treated him the same, although justified? Still, she could've handled the situation much better than to go off on him like that, justified or not.

Enough, she thought. Determined not to dwell on things she couldn't change, she locked her doors, turned off the lights in the living room and kitchen, and walked into her bedroom. She flipped the light switch and admired the work the contractors had done to fix the tree damage. A faint hint of fresh paint enveloped her. It didn't bother her; instead, she likened it to the scent of a new car. It reminded her of change, new beginnings. She didn't know how positive her changes would be, but she had to focus on the good that happened in her life. It kept her going.

With a new resolve, she changed into her nighty,

turned the covers on her bed, and reached for the romance novel on her nightstand. *Things would get better. They had to*, she thought.

CHAPTER FIFTEEN

*S*aturday, Jenna spent most of her time catching up on household chores and doing a quick grocery run. With her shoulder still sore and contractors working on her house, there had been no point in doing any other chores last week beside keeping on top of her dishes and sweeping the main traffic areas. Now that her house looked presentable again, she stood back with a satisfied smile to admire her work. *Everything will be fine,* she told herself, then took a quick shower. She was looking forward to her well-overdue and deserved girls' night out, and she was determined to have a good time.

A car horn honked, and after a quick check in the mirror, Jenna grabbed her purse and locked her door on the way out. "Hi, Beth," she said after skipping to her friend's car. "Thanks for picking me up." She sat down in the passenger seat.

"You deserve to be pampered. You've done so much for me in the last few weeks, and this is the least I can do."

"Oh, stop it! You stepped right up when I was incapacitated. We would've had to shut down shop if it wasn't for you, Willow, and Clarissa."

Beth's cheeks took on a slight shade of pink. "You know I'd do anything for you," she said. "Either way, let's get going. I'm starving. Anna called me earlier and said she'll meet us at the Sappy Pine." Beth pulled out of the driveway.

"I can't wait," Jenna said. "We hadn't done a girls' night in ages."

"It's been long overdue," Beth agreed.

A few minutes later, they arrived downtown at the bar. Anna was already waiting by the entrance, checking her phone. She looked up and her face brightened as she waved at them.

Beth pulled into a vacant parking space. "Let's forget all about work and the crazy doc. We're going to have a fun, worry-free weekend."

"Deal! This is our night," Jenna agreed, and they got out of the car.

Anna shoved her phone into her back pocket of her jeans and rushed over to embrace them in a tight group hug. "It's been so long since we've had an evening out together," she said, then flashed a deck of cards. "I bought a fresh deck just for this occasion."

The girls laughed.

"You didn't mark them, did you?" Beth asked.

"Nope, still in the wrapper," Anna said. "Let's go inside."

They entered the bar and sat in a booth far enough from the speakers where they could still hear each other over the classic rock playing in the background.

"What can I get you to start out with?" the waitress asked.

The girls looked at each other and giggled. "That'll be wine, like the good old times," Anna answered. "A bottle of Merlot and three glasses. And I almost forgot, a glass of water for each of us. Otherwise, this will be a short night."

Beth smiled. "Good call. I'm afraid I've turned into a lightweight over the last couple of years."

"Can you also bring us some buffalo wings and potato skins as an appetizer for the table to share?" Jenna asked. "Knowing us, it'll take a minute to figure out what we want for dinner."

The menu was fairly limited, but for bar food it wasn't that bad, and Jenna always had a hard time picking between the Rockin' Boat Fish & Chips Basket, the Rock 'n' Roll Burger Basket, or the Mixed Tape Sampler Platter with quesadilla wedges, mozzarella sticks, and two chicken tenders. All of the choices were good.

After the waitress brought them their wine, Anna raised her glass. "To enduring friendship!"

"To enduring friendship," Jenna and Beth repeated in unison as they clinked glasses.

Anna set down her glass again, glanced down at the table, and outlined the heart with the initials AW and JM carved into the wood with her finger. "Remember when Jason carved that heart into the table with his pock-etknife?" Anna said with a smile, her eyes sparkling.

"I do," Jenna said. "He said he'd never stop loving you."

"And look where you are today?" Beth said. "A happy couple again."

"Speaking of men, what are your guys doing tonight?" Jenna asked.

"Kevin is hanging out with Sean today, believe it or not," Beth said while studying her one page menu. "When they first met, they couldn't stand each other, but now they get along splendid. He said something about them helping a friend on a project."

Anna looked at her, confused. "Hmm, Jason said the same to me." She shrugged her shoulders. "Must be some big project they are working on. Maybe they are building a deck for someone."

"Who knows," Jenna said. "I have to tell you, though, I was thankful for all the help I got after the tornado. That's why I love this town so much. When someone is in trouble or needs a hand, the people of Magnolia Hill always come together and support you through it."

"I agree," Anna said. "When I came back home after living in Colorado for over a decade, everyone, or let's say almost everyone, was happy to see me and made me feel welcome again. Except for Gracie. Remember she was my worst nightmare in high school? She has come a long way and surprised the heck out of me when she came apologizing the day Jason proposed to me."

"I do remember that," Jenna said, nodding. "She did a complete one-eighty and turned her life around. Good for her."

"Let's hope it lasts," Anna said. "I never liked her, but now that she's getting help, she's changed so much for the better." Anna shrugged her shoulders. "For a lack of a better term, I'd say she acts… more human."

Jenna nodded. "That may be true, but it's still awkward trying to have a conversation with her. I saw Gracie at the grocery store the other day, and neither one of us had anything to say. The silence was painful, so I told her it was good to see her and went about my business."

Beth took a sip of her wine. "Give her some time. She's new at this acting civil and not snarling thing."

The waitress brought the wings and potato skins to the table, took their dinner order, and rushed off again.

"So, Jenna," Anna started. "Are you going to keep the new line of cupcakes going? My mom has been raving about them all week long."

Beth shushed her. "We're here to have fun, not talk about work."

"It's okay, Beth. I haven't decided yet," Jenna admitted. "Considering after what had happened yesterday, I'm on the fence. It's tempting, because they sell very well, but if Cody has his way, I'll be out of business soon and will have to work at the diner again."

"But look at all the support we have from the community. I doubt he can shut us down," Beth said. "Besides, it would be crazy not to keep them going. They are a hit!"

Jenna sighed. "I know. It's just that continuing the low-carb line would be like letting Cody have his way. It's like giving up or selling out, depends on from what angle you want to look at it."

"Okay, so since we're looking at angles," Anna said, "have you considered that offering and expanding the Doctor-Approved line could considerably increase your profits? And"—she paused for good measure—"should there be any legal issues, you can prove that you're showing goodwill by going above and beyond to meet him in the middle."

"I like that spin," Beth added. "Actually, this would be

a win for everyone. You keep our customers happy by giving them an alternative, you make more money so we can upgrade some of the appliances you've been holding off on, and Doc Walker can save the world, or whatever it is he wants to do." Beth clapped her hands together, then reached her arms out in the air. "There you go, everyone's happy."

"I'll think about it," Jenna said and helped herself to another chicken wing. "Remember, we're not here to think about Doc Walker. This is our night. No guys allowed!"

"That's right, no guys allowed," Anna echoed.

After the women polished off their meals, and the wait-ress cleared their table, Anna pulled out the new deck of cards with cover art featuring an elegant bottle of red wine with a partially filled glass next to it. "I thought this deck was appropriate for this occasion," she added as she pulled on the tab to remove the clear wrapper, pulled the cards out of the box, then shuffled the deck.

"Before we get started"—Beth stood—"I need to visit the ladies' room."

"Me, too," Jenna added. "Can you deal while we're gone, Anna?"

"Sure, I promise I won't cheat," she said with a wink.

When Jenna and Beth returned. Anna had already dealt the cards and stacked them on the table for them.

Jenna scooted into the corner of their booth.

"Oh, no. What are they doing here?" Beth said, her jaw open as she was about to slide into the booth.

Anna turned around. "What the…?"

Jenna watched Jason, Kevin, and Sean entered the bar, followed by none other than Cody, who looked extremely uncomfortable, at best. Suddenly, the large room closed in on her as claustrophobia set in. No, she could not be in the same room as him. Not tonight.

"When Kevin said he was helping a friend, he didn't mention that friend was Doc Walker," Beth said.

"Nope, same here. Jason didn't mention him either."

The men looked as if they got caught with their hands in the cookie jar and were about to bolt.

"Not so fast," Beth said, stomping toward them. "Why are you hanging out with *him*?" she said, pointing at Cody.

Kevin raked his hand through his hair and shifted his weight to his other leg. "Uh, we helped Cody set up a new obstacle and then did a quick workout. We were just finishing up with a beer. I thought you guys went to Jenna's?"

"Nope, I never said that. I picked her up. And work out? You?" Beth said with a laugh, then sobered. "Are you aware that this guy wants to shut down the bakery?"

"It's not like that, Beth," Sean said.

"Stay out of this!" Beth shouted. "My job is on the line, and you're fraternizing with the enemy?"

"He has a nice ninja setup in his backyard, though," Kevin admitted.

"You gals should really listen to what Cody has to say," Sean said. "It's not what it looks like."

Jenna and Anna joined Beth and stood their ground with their arms crossed. Then Jenna made a mistake she immediately regretted. She made eye contact with Cody. Anger, guilt, empathy, and a whole other slew of emotions ambushed her all at once. It took all the effort she could muster to look away. "Beth, I've got to go. Can you drive me home?"

"Don't let them spoil our fun," Beth said.

"Please?" Jenna pleaded, barely audible.

Her friend nodded. "Of course." She then pointed at Kevin. "We're not done yet."

"And neither are we." Anna glared at Jason.

The men made a U-turn and scrambled out the door.

"Thanks, girls, for having my back," Jenna said. "I really didn't mean to get you all dragged into this fight."

"Don't worry," Anna said. "Us girls have to stick together!"

"Thank you," she said, fighting to hold back her tears.

~

Two more weeks went by, and Cody had just finished another one of his morning workouts on his ninja playground. He decided that laying low would be an excellent strategy for now, especially around Jenna as she had made it clear that she didn't want to talk to or even be in the same room with him. With his luck, he'd run from her property with icing knives, for a lack of a better term, sticking out of his back. Even though some of his patients came around, and he was thankful that Jenna still offered the low-carb cupcakes in her shop, he was not happy with the situation. It bothered him that there was a divide between them. They could've had such a wonderful work relationship, and if he had pushed his luck in a more positive way instead of letting his laser-narrow focus destroy what could've been a wonderful thing, they could've spent evenings on his porch together after a nice workout. But, of course, he messed that up all by himself, and he wasn't sure how to undo the damage—if that was even possible. She was so close, yet it felt as if they were thousands of miles apart from each other.

No matter how hard he tried to distract himself with workouts, projects, or studying medical journals, Jenna stayed on his mind. And every day without fail, something would remind him of his foolish mistakes. Yes, he had made many, and by the looks of it, he hadn't learned from any of them. Instead, he made things worse. It killed him seeing her when she wrote her daily sales on her chalk sidewalk sign in front of her shop, or when she got into her car and drove home—not that he was stalking her, he just noticed movement from his peripheral vision outside of his office window. What's worse, he also had to drive past her house every time he went to town, which was pure torture, especially when her car was in the driveway. What he really wanted to do was stop by and see her. Of course, he knew better than that.

This whole thing had to end, and he had to figure out how he could win her trust back. Even if it took baby steps and years to make things right, he owed it to her, the town, and himself. Magnolia Hill was his home now, and he had to do his part to be accepted back into the community, if he ever had been.

Goosebumps appeared on his arms from the chill of the November air. Rubbing his forearms, he went inside, showered, and made some breakfast. He cracked a couple of eggs into one side of a hot cast-iron frying pan with a teaspoon worth of bacon grease for flavoring. On the side he browned some chopped onions, freshly pressed garlic, and a few rings of miniature bell peppers. The aroma of his hearty breakfast filled his kitchen and made his mouth water. He spread the sizzling veggies around with a small spatula, and already the onions began to caramelize, giving them a nice brown edge. While he waited for his breakfast to cook, he seasoned his eggs and pulled out a medium-sized plate and a fork. When his sunny side up eggs were firm enough for his taste, he separated the two eggs that had run together with his spatula and transferred the first one onto his plate.

The second one seemed to have a mind of its own and clung to the pan. "Darn it," he said. Despite the years of faithful seasoning his cast-iron cookware, it wasn't cooperating today. He shoved the spatula under the browned edge of the egg closest to the center, then with mini pushes freed the egg.

Proud of his cooking skills, Cody picked up the plate and lifted the egg out of the pan. However, his bubble of bliss burst when the egg-yolk went top-heavy on one side and slid off his spatula, grazing the edge of his plate and hitting the floor runny-yolk down.

"No! Darn it all again!" he grumbled as he looked at the mess by his feet. He wasn't sure if he should be sad about losing part of his breakfast or mad for having to clean up the yolk that ran into the grout of his kitchen's tile flooring. Maybe both.

Not wanting to fight with dried-up egg goo later, he wet a wad of paper towels, picked up the egg, and scrubbed the yolk out of the grout. By the time he got to his breakfast, his food was only lukewarm. At this point, he didn't care anymore. He just hoped that this wasn't a sign of how his day would go.

Mostly satisfied from his meal, Cody poured another cup of coffee with a splash of heavy cream and pulled out a notepad from his junk drawer to make a list of what all he had done wrong since his arrival in Magnolia Hill and how he could redeem himself. He began with all his mistakes.

- *Threatening to close down Jenna's shop*

- *Attempting to file a complaint with the Chamber & BBB*

- *Writing that awful article*

- *Being at war with Miriam Sue, although she deserved it*

- *Causing arguments between Jason and Kevin and their better halves*

- *Overwhelming my patients with strict dietary rules*

- *Whatever else I screwed up*

The longer he thought about it, he realized his actions affected most people in town to some extent—and not in a good way. Yes, he had come to Magnolia Hill to make a difference, but this wasn't the kind of difference he had in mind.

Cody picked up the pen again and made a separate list of what he wanted instead.

- *A partnership between the practice and Jenna's shop (and maybe more)*

- *Help my patients heal, but in a way that's doable for them*

- *Have a good relationship with the people in this town, something I didn't have time for in my old job*

- *Grow my ninja playground and work the legal piece to allow others in the community to use it*

When he couldn't think of anything else, he set down his pen next to the notepad and leaned back in his chair with a smile. Reading over this last list, he realized that his priorities had been all wrong. It was all about community.

It always had been. A warm, fuzzy feeling spread throughout his body as he wrote down the word in large bold letters across the paper and circled it several times. Yes, whatever he did from here on out, he had to keep this word in mind. Cody had the right idea when he arrived in Magnolia Hill, but how he went about it achieved the exact opposite. Now, with a new sense of clarity, he knew what he had to do.

Cody tore the sheet of paper with the lists off his notepad, laid it to the side, and with a fresh page in front of him, began brainstorming. He wrote four words spread out on the page and circled each of them. The words were: *Jenna, Patients, Newspaper, Playground.* Instead of dread, excitement spread from his chest to his fingertips, and he could barely keep up with jotting down the ideas that popped into his mind.

When he ran out of room, he decided it was time for action. He picked up his phone and dialed a now familiar number from his recent calls list.

"Hello, Cody," the female voice answered.

"Hi Kristen," he said, his voice cracking with excitement.

CHAPTER SIXTEEN

By Monday, Cody was as nervous as a teenager asking a girl to prom. He was going to talk to Jenna later, and it could either go well or turn out to be an absolute disaster. He preferred the first outcome, but he couldn't blame her if she didn't want to be a part of what he was about to propose to her.

After he saw his last patient before lunch, he picked up one of the flyers he had handed out to his diabetic patients and brought it with him. "Wish me luck, Twyla," he said to his receptionist.

She gave him an unsure smile. "You'll need it," she said. "As mad as she is, she might kick you head-first out of her bakery. I give you fifty seconds." She pointed at her watch.

"Not even a minute, huh?" he said with a mock frown. "You don't have much confidence this will work, do you?"

"Nope. Not really," she said. "Good luck, anyway. I'm rooting for ya!"

"Thanks, Twyla. I need it." At least he was on good

terms with his staff again. It took a few days for them to come around after he came clean with them at the staff meeting that dreadful day, but Cody was thankful they understood. And because of them, not all of his patients had abandoned him.

Cody headed out the door, his heart beating up to his throat in overtime. He took a deep, calming breath in an attempt to slow his heart, but without success. When he reached the Cherry-on-Top glass door, he paused for a moment to focus on the task ahead, then took another deep breath and opened the door.

Willow, today with green hair, stood behind the counter.

It didn't take an ability to read minds to know what she was thinking. "Hi Willow," he said to break the ice.

"Hello, Dr. Walker," she said, then turned. "I'll go get Jenna, unless you're here to actually buy something this time."

"Thank you," he said. "I will do that too. Make it four low-carb cupcakes for the clinic, please." Then he waited. He looked down at his medical alert bracelet and spun it around his wrist, reminding himself why he was here—the health of the community.

Jenna walked out of the kitchen, drying her hands on her apron. "What?" she said with an undertone even the densest person would understand was not welcoming.

"Before you throw me to the curb, please hear me out. I'm putting together a diabetes talk for the people of Magnolia Hill and our neighboring towns, and I want you to cater treats," he rattled off, pushing the flyer in front of her before she could say anything else.

She picked up the flyer and propped her other hand on

her waist. "Why would I do you any favors after you told the entire town I was going to kill them with my sweets?"

She didn't rip up the flyer and throw the paper shreds back at him. He considered that a good start. "I want to give back to our community by teaching patients and their loved ones about diabetes and how to make positive life-style changes without increasing their medications. That evening will be one of many free educational events in the works," he said with a tentative smile. "Twyla reserved the conference room at the Chamber for Tuesday evening next week, and we're setting up some low-carb options for everyone to try. Your cupcakes, I'm sure, will be the first to disappear," he said, then raked his hand through his hair. "Please say yes. If you don't want to cater, I could pick them up, too. Of course, I'll pay extra for all the trouble, if you can deliver them. I really want you to be part of this."

She looked up at him, then averted her gaze and pushed the flyer back at him. "Sorry, I can't."

"Think about it?" he asked and slowly pushed the flyer back at her. "All I ask from you is to consider it. Don't do it for me; do it for the people of Magnolia Hill. Just because we have our differences doesn't mean everyone has to miss out on trying your new line of cupcakes." He waited for a response, but none come. "Please?"

She sighed. "Okay, I'll think about it, but don't get your hopes up."

He cupped her hand with both of his, then pulled them off as soon as he realized what he was doing. "Thank you, Jenna," he said. "I'll check back by the end of the week if I don't hear from you by then."

"Again, don't count on it," she said.

Just the fact that she talked to him was a success in his

book. His proposal went better than he had expected. "Whatever you decide, I'm fine with it," he said with a grin, "but I really think your cupcakes will fly off the snack table, based on the initial feedback I got from my patients." Cody noticed some movement by the kitchen door in his peripheral vision. He looked over and caught two heads disappearing behind the frame—one was green. "Bye, Willow and Beth!"

There was some commotion and whispering, then they stepped out into the shop. "Sorry for eavesdropping," Beth said.

"Well, ladies, I better head back over to the practice," he said. "If you could box me up those four wonderful Doctor-Approved cupcakes... I heard they were healthy and taste like heaven. My staff would strangle me if I came all the way over here and not bring them any goodies back."

"Willow, can you take care of that?" Jenna said and disappeared in the kitchen.

"Thank you, Jenna," he called after her.

"Wow, you lasted longer than I thought," Twyla said, eyeballing the box in his hands when he got back to his clinic. "I must admit, I underestimated you when it comes to talking to women."

"No, Twyla. I wouldn't call it that. All I did was figure out what was important—and the people of Magnolia Hill are just that."

❧

*T*he week flew by, and the demand for the new cupcakes was higher than Jenna could've dreamed of. While Willow was out delivering pies and cupcakes to Mamaw's Diner, Jenna kept an eye out for customers. Beth was decorating another batch for the afternoon rush. "Those look great," Jenna said. "I think we discovered your hidden talent."

Beth blushed. "It was hidden alright." She topped the last cupcake of the batch with a final dot of whipped cream and stood back with a satisfied smile that brightened her face. "Thank you for believing in me and giving me a chance. I always wanted to learn how to bake, but I never had the time. The few occasions I tried, I was always missing an ingredient or two, and we all know how that usually turns out."

"Well, I'm so proud of you, Beth," Jenna said. "Way to go with stepping out of your comfort zone and learning something new."

Jenna heard the shop door open, and Maggie entered the bakery. "Hello Jenna," she said. "I just came from my appointment with Dr. Walker, and I'm here to pick up my usual treat. Today is special, and I want to celebrate that my blood sugar values are improving."

"That's wonderful news. Congratulations. How are you feeling?" Jenna asked.

"Much better, actually. Not so tired and jittery all the time like I used to be. I seem to have more energy, which comes in handy with the holidays just around the corner when people have more time for crafts."

"I've seen a lot more cars parked in front of your store since Anna and Ashleigh helped you refresh your craft shop," Jenna said. "I'm so happy you could turn things around again."

"I'm forever grateful. If it wasn't for my girls coming back home to Magnolia Hill, I would've retired last summer. But now, people come out of the woodworks wanting to finish their knitting and crocheting projects they had tucked away decades ago. It's like everyone remembered how relaxing needle crafts are."

"I used to love knitting when I was younger," Jenna said with a sigh, "but now my hours are so long, I can hardly find time to be still for a moment. Sometimes I wish I was a teenager again. Willow tells me you have a lot of high schoolers coming to your classes."

"I've got Ashleigh and Sarah to thank for that. If it wasn't for the girls making those teeny-bopper friendship bracelets and starting to offer classes on how to make them, it would've never happened. It was like a chain reaction. Kids worked on their crafts, then moms remembered they had a project in the closet they had been meaning to finish. Adding the comfy craft nook in our shop where everyone can work on their projects and socialize at the same time has been the perfect touch."

"I'm so excited for you, Maggie. And having Anna back in town is just what I needed. It's been good to have the old gang back together again," Jenna said. "So, how many cupcakes would you like today?"

"I'll take two of the Doctor-Approved cupcakes, one for me and one for Anna. She's off work today, so she's helping at the shop. And I want one of those with the gummy fish on the icing for Ashleigh when she gets home from school. What did you call these, Hurricane Gerard Blasts?" she asked.

"They are called Hurricane Caramel Swirl cupcakes," she said.

"Yes, one of them," Maggie said. "So, do you have plans on expanding these low-carb versions of your original recipes? I really would love something like the birthday cake one or the strawberry swirl cupcakes so I can alternate them."

"You might be able to talk me into it," Jenna said and winked at her friend's mom.

"If anyone can make the healthy version taste almost more heavenly than the sugary cupcakes, it's you," Maggie said. "Besides, I don't think Doc Walker is all that bad as people make him out to be," she added. "Miriam Sue wrote an apology for printing that dreadful article, and I think our doc is coming around. Have you read today's paper yet?"

"I have not," Jenna said.

"Well, it's worth a read. I'm going to see what his diabetes talk is all about next week, and I heard from several of my knitting club ladies that they are coming, too." She then paid for her treats and headed back to her craft shop.

Jenna wondered what that article was all about. It swayed Maggie to trust Cody again, so there must be something to it. Although she couldn't imagine it would have the same effect on her. That article last week was the straw that broke the camel's back for her. He'd have to try mighty hard to convince her to trust him again, and she wasn't even sure that she ever could.

When Willow returned from her delivery, her high green pigtails bopped from side to side as she walked around the counter. "Roberta at the diner said she needs more of those low-fat doctor cupcakes everyone's been asking about for dessert." She rolled her eyes. "I don't know how many times I have to tell her that they are low carb. Either way, people are asking for them."

"Thank you, Willow," Jenna said. "You're doing a wonderful job, and I can't say it enough that we're so lucky to have you work here."

Willow smiled, then lowered her head. "I'm just helping customers, keeping the area clean, and making the delivery runs, that's all."

Beth joined them from the back. "You don't *just* help out. Before you started, we'd been struggling to keep our heads above water. It was just too much work for only two of us. With your help, and Clarissa's baked goodies on consignment, we can focus on making more cupcakes and other special orders."

"I'm glad to pitch in wherever I can," Willow said with a slight blush shading her cheeks a faint pink, then turned away. "I better make more Doctor-Approved labels for the next batch."

Speaking of the doctor, Jenna couldn't get that article out of her mind. What was in the paper that Maggie wanted her to read? She knew she would not get any peace of mind until she'd get a hold of a copy of the Magnolia Hill Herald. "I'll be right back," Jenna said and grabbed her fleece. "Keep an eye out for the cupcakes in the oven, will ya, Beth?"

When Jenna stepped out of the bakery, a cool breeze hit her face, and despite her fleece, goosebumps popped up on her arms. She had to hurry, or she'd turn into an icicle. Jenna considered her choices. She could walk across the street and grab a paper from the newspaper dispenser outside of Cody's practice or walk down a block to Mamaw's Diner. A cold raindrop landed on her face and ran down her cheek. She really didn't want to chance running into Cody, so walking to the diner was her first preference. But when she looked up to the sky, and gray ominous clouds threatened to burst wide open any moment, she reluctantly opted for crossing the street in hopes Cody was busy seeing patients.

She waited for a pickup truck to pass, then ran across the street, pulled the door of the newspaper dispenser, and grabbed one of the thin papers. As she let the spring door snap shut again, the door behind her opened.

"Until next month, Mr. Coleman," a familiar voice said.

Out of reflex, she turned toward the voice, and her eyes met with Cody's. He was about to say something, when, as if on cue, the sky opened up, and rain poured down on her. "Sorry, gotta go," she said and ran with her paper tucked under her arm across the street and back to her bakery.

Not bothering to take off her fleece, she unfolded the paper and laid it flat on the counter.

The headline read: *A Letter from the Community Doctor.*

Jenna skimmed down and saw Miriam Sue's apology that the author had retracted original article prior to publication. It also said that the article was printed in error and it should've never happened.

So the rumors were true, Jenna thought. He didn't mean to publish that piece. Yet, it still hurt inside when she thought about how his intent had been to shut her down.

Her eyes wandered back to the article.

"Read it out loud," Beth said.

Jenna cleared her throat.

Dear Reader,

I came to Magnolia Hill for several reasons: to escape the stress of a relentless city life, for my own health reasons, and most importantly, to help as many patients as possible to get and stay well. At the beginning, I may have been a bit too focused on my own goal, and instead of considering each and every one in your town with separate needs, I have been too rigid in my approach. Instead of helping, I alienated many of you. I understand that now and have realized where I went wrong. When I took over the practice, I promised Dr. Porter that I would get to know his patients—that would be you—and take the time it took to treat them. Instead of listening to what your individual needs and life circumstances were, I pushed a one-way only approach on you. For that, I'm sorry. My other mistake was misjudging some members of your community and treating them unfairly because of my own bias. For that I'm truly sorry, too. I have much to learn yet, but in the meantime, I want to offer my services as an educator on anything health-related you might be interested in. My goal is to get to know your wonderful community and your unique needs. I want to start off Tuesday evening at 6 o'clock at the Chamber of Commerce with a diabetes presentation followed by an open discussion. Anyone interested is invited. I want to hold these types of events regularly for you in hopes to get to know you better and be of better service to you.

Jenna sighed. "He sounds like he is trying to make up for his mistakes."

"Do you think he means it?" Beth asked.

Willow's pigtails bopped again as she nodded. "I think he does."

Beth turned to Jenna. "Maybe you should give him another chance. Make some cupcakes for his event and go from there."

Jenna wanted to believe in him as much as they did, but she'd been burned too many times. She wasn't sure if she could trust him not to blind-side her again. "I don't know."

"Well, I still think we should cater," Beth said. "It's a win-win situation for all of us."

"Seriously, Jenna, what do we have to lose?" Willow added.

Jenna thought for a moment. Other than their personal difference, she didn't have any good reasons why they shouldn't. "Okay, ladies. What are you waiting for? We've got recipes to convert by next week."

CHAPTER SEVENTEEN

*O*n Tuesday evening, Jenna, Beth, and Willow packed a dozen containers of the new Doctor-Approved line of mini-sample cupcakes into crates.

Butterflies fluttered about in the pit of Jenna's stomach. What if the guests didn't like the new flavors? Their converted recipes had been top-secret, and the girls decided they would surprise everyone with the grand reveal at the event tonight. What she was more nervous about, though, was Cody. This was strictly a professional arrangement. There was no reason for her hands to shake. *It's just business,* she reminded herself.

"I'll grab another handful of the business cards," Willow said and wrapped a rubber band around the stack she had picked up from the counter.

Jenna ran through her checklist on her clipboard for the hundredth time:

- *Cupcakes*
- *Display trays*
- *Table cloth*

- Decoration

- Napkins

- Business cards, thanks to Willow

"I think we have everything," Jenna said, grabbing the last bag to put in the company vehicle.

They drove the short stretch to the Chamber down the street.

When they arrived, Cody stood by the door, dressed in jeans, a dress shirt, and a jacket. He saw them pull up, then rushed toward them.

He cleans up nicely, Jenna thought, and the flutters returned. No. She was only here to reveal her new cupcake flavors, nothing else.

"Hi Jenna," he greeted her, "Ladies. Thank you for catering tonight. Let me help you carry some of this stuff in," he said, and without waiting, picked up the plastic container with the display stands. "Just follow me to the conference room," he said.

As Jenna entered the conference room, she stopped dead in her tracks. That woman who Cody was so cozy with lately was standing in front of a laptop pulling up a slide presentation on the projector screen.

In an instant, all hopes for a nice evening had evaporated. Her presence alone made Jenna's stomach twist and bend in a slow churning motion.

"Jenna, meet Kristin. She's a registered dietitian in Savannah," he said. "Jenna is the creator of these wonderful cupcakes," he explained, pointing at the table in the back where Willow and Beth already arranged a few of the sample cupcakes.

The woman reached out her hand. "Nice to meet you, Jenna."

Reluctantly, Jenna reciprocated. The woman's hand was cool to the touch. "Same here," she replied in a not so enthusiastic tone. "I better help set up in the back," Jenna said. "Please excuse me." Not only was Cody spending a lot of time with her, now she also was a speaker at his save the community event. It was because of her that Cody had been so distant after their baking adventure. There was no doubt in her mind. With a polite smile, she turned and joined Beth and Willow at the snack table.

Jenna knew it was rude of her to walk away, but she couldn't stomach being around that woman much longer, as much as she couldn't stand being close to Cody. There were just too many reminders of how gullible she had been the last few weeks. She didn't need any more of that dull, lingering pain in her chest telling her she should've listened to her gut.

"What is she doing here?" Beth asked, emphasizing the *she*.

"She's some sort of dietician," Jenna said. "Maybe she's his slide-flipper."

Beth chuckled, then arranged a stack of small, square, pastel-colored napkins next to the mini-cupcakes.

"What do you think?" Willow asked, motioning at the beautifully decorated display in a Vanna White fashion.

"Great job, ladies," Jenna said. "And thank you for helping me set up. I couldn't have done any better myself." She smiled. "You ladies are both free to leave, if you want. I got it from here."

"Are you sure?" Willow asked. "I was going to check on my grandma tonight but wanted to make sure you're good here."

"I'm fine. Go visit your grandma, and I'll see you again in the morning," Jenna said.

"Thank you," Willow said, waving goodbye to them as she left.

Beth nudged Jenna's side and leaned in. "So, what do you think, you know, about her?"

"She actually seems nice, but I just can't..." Jenna replied with a sour taste in her mouth.

"I totally get it," Beth said. "I can stay through the event and clean up the table afterwards, if you want to leave."

"It's tempting," Jenna said, "but I'm the owner of the business, and I wouldn't feel right leaving you here doing all my work. Besides, I'm sure Kevin is already at home waiting for you."

Beth gave her a reproachful look. "I really don't mind. Trust me, I can see it in your eyes that you don't want to do this."

"You're right; I don't. But this is my bakery. If I leave you here by yourself, there's going to be a lot of chatter in town tomorrow about why I wasn't there for the big reveal." She caught Cody's gaze from the other end of the room, but she looked away.

"True." Beth grabbed her purse. "But if you change your mind, call me, okay? I'm only a hop and a skip away."

"Go home and spend time with your honey-bunny," she said. "All that's left to do after the event is to take our serving dishes back to the bakery. I'm pretty certain I can handle that much on my own."

"Okay, then. I'm heading out," Beth said. "Good luck with the cupcakes."

Little by little, the room filled with locals.

"Bless you for making my favorite cupcake so I can eat it," Maggie said, taking one of the birthday cake samples.

Jenna waited with bated breath for any sign of approval or disapproval.

Maggie closed her eyes as she bit into it. "Thank you, thank you, thank you," she said. "These are wonderful. I used to sneak some of your cupcakes every so often when Ashleigh had some left over, but with these, I can have a treat and not feel guilty about it." She licked a dab of icing off her lip. "They are also very filling. After eating one of your healthy cupcakes, I can't even think of having another. And you know me…"

Jenna laughed. "It's the almond flour that makes it more dense and more satisfying."

"Well, I don't care what's in it. All I know is that I love it," Maggie said.

"Love what, Mom?" Anna came up behind her and rested her chin on Maggie's shoulder.

"The new doctor cupcakes Jenna made." Maggie picked up a chocolate mini-cupcake and held it in front of Anna's lips. "Open up."

"Wow," Anna said once she got her words back. "I'm going to sit in the back and help you guard the table."

"Be nice, Anna." Jenna wagged her finger at her. "You have to learn how to share."

"Not those magic cupcakes," her friend replied.

The lights dimmed in the room.

"All right, everybody. Let's get started," Cody said from the stage area in the front of the room. "Thank you all for coming to today's diabetes talk. This is going to be one of many events where we begin with an educational session and then follow up with answering questions you may have about the topic. In addition, I want to get some small groups going at the practice where you can ask questions and exchange recipes, among other things. This will be on a smaller scale. Most important, you are not alone, and as a community, we can support each other, even if we sometimes don't feel so well."

Jenna took a seat on a black metal folding chair next to her table. It wasn't comfortable by any means, but it would do. Scanning the room, she had to admit that he had a good turnout, considering the whole blunder with the paper. She also had to give him credit for trying to make things right with her and the people of this town.

"But first, I want to introduce you to Kristen McMillan," he said, and the woman stood and joined him in the front. "She is a registered dietitian and has an office near the Medical Center in Savannah." He smiled. "Kristen agreed to help me with the food portion of this talk. Her husband, Steve, is sitting right here in the front row, so don't forget to say hello to him later."

Husband? She was married? Was she wrong all this time? Jenna closed her eyes. How foolish she had been.

"And don't forget about the baby!" Steve called out.

Kristen gently rubbed her small belly.

A baby? How could she have missed that fact? Was she so wrapped up in her own anger that she didn't notice that small baby bump? Jenna never felt so ashamed in her entire life.

"But before we dive into today's topic, let me tell you a short story of why we are here today." The first slide on the projector screen showed a picture of two young doctors. "This was me fifteen years ago, right after medical school with my best friend Scott. We both wanted to save the world. Turns out, he saved mine. You see, I was an overworked physician in a busy practice in Atlanta. We only had ten minutes to spend with each patient to keep up with our schedule—which was not even close enough to what I needed to treat them appropriately. Burned out, addicted to sugar and bread, and no time to take care of myself, my body couldn't handle the stress anymore. Six months ago, I woke up on a stretcher rolling down the halls of the Emory ER. Scott was the one who told me I had a heart attack, and if I didn't change my life, next time I wouldn't be so lucky. He also broke the news to me that I was a diabetic. It didn't surprise me with all the pastries and sweets I ate. I just couldn't stop. But living in denial was less painful than dealing with the rest of my miserable life."

He clicked to the next slide with a picture of a much chubbier version of himself. Gasps filled the room. "This was me a few months before my heart attack. Hard to believe I was giving my patients dietary advice," he said with a chuckle. "Scott had told me in no uncertain terms that I had to change my life if I wanted to live another year. He also reminded me of what used to be important to me in med school. Why was I doing this? My answer was to save as many patients as possible. But first I had to save myself. While recovering from my stent surgery and getting my affairs in Atlanta in order, I went on a mission to read up on the newest research on how to first fix myself and then use that new knowledge to help my patients. I've been there. And I want to help you. That's why we're here. I pledge to you that I will continue studying cutting edge research to help you and your families improve the quality of your life, if you let me. It will not be all boring and sending you off with a sack full of pills after appointments. Who said that you can't have a little fun in life?" Cody's gaze stopped at Jenna. "And if you give me another chance, I promise I will do all that I can so that you will get to spend many, many precious years creating memories with your family."

~

*J*enna's heart melted on the spot. He spoke to her. Was he asking her for forgiveness and promising to spend the rest of his life with her? No. It couldn't be. She was wrong to assume he and Kristen had a thing going on. Now, she imagined he promised her the world. But what if?

She could feel the palpitations drumming up a storm in her chest. Jenna didn't know he'd been through so much. From the get-go, she had misjudged him. She had thought of him as an arrogant, rich city doctor who would not even give her the time of day. Because of her bias, she couldn't see the person who hid behind that protective wall he had built around him, even after she had caught a glimpse of the gentle and caring man he was inside.

Jenna now understood. His passion to save people got off on a wonky start, but all he wanted to do was save the world. That didn't excuse his behavior, but she also understood how hard it must've been for someone addicted to food to work across the street of a bakery. She would've been cranky, too, especially if she saw the people she wanted to help run straight into the lion's den. She got it now. Her vibes had been right all along.

He glanced at her from the side of the room as Kristin was giving her presentation.

She could tell that he wanted to break away and talk to her, like he wanted to when he helped bring the cupcakes into the conference room, but for now he had to stay put.

"So that wraps up my presentation," Kristen said. "Let's use the rest of our time to answer questions you might have for me or Dr. Walker."

Jenna suppressed a chuckle when she saw Cody jump and rush to join Kristen's side in the front of the room. The audience's interest in the topic surprised her and several hands went up after they had answered each question.

"Go ahead, Maggie," Cody said, nodding at her.

"So, I can have as many of those Doctor-Approved cupcakes as I want?" she asked.

Anna shushed her. "No, Mom. I told you."

"Good question," Cody said. "But before I go into any detail, I want to say thank you to Jenna from the Cherry on Top Cupcake Shop. As you know, she worked diligently on creating the best low-carb cupcakes on the market for our diabetic patients and anyone else, for that matter. And as a surprise, she brought in new samples of the Doctor-Approved low-carb cupcake line."

Jenna stood and pointed at her display.

"If you haven't tried them yet," Cody continued, "feel free to grab a couple samples on the way out later on. Jenna, would you like to say a few words about your new creations?"

Jenna flushed and her hands tingled, then became numb. She was terrified of public speaking. "Uh." Her mind went blank.

"It's okay, I didn't mean to put you on the spot," he said.

Get yourself together, she thought. "Oh, no. It's fine." It wasn't, but if she wanted to get excitement over her cupcakes going, she had to say something.

"Chocolate," Anna whispered, pointing at the cupcakes.

"Oh, yes. As you can see, we converted some of our bestselling cupcakes into low-carb versions, so you don't have to miss out. We have the Death by Chocolate, Strawberry Swirl, and the Birthday Cake cupcakes added to our Doctor-Approved assortment in addition to the Lemon Cheesecake flavor many of you have already tried. We also have some other delicious ideas in the works, so keep coming back to see us when you're in town."

The crowd clapped.

Jenna quickly sat before anyone could ask questions she might not have the answer to. She didn't mind talking to her customers face to face—she knew everybody in the room—but standing in the spotlight had always been a terrifying experience for her. That fear of standing in front of people and drawing a blank—or worse, making an utter fool of herself—was a nightmare.

Anna gave her the thumbs up.

"Thank you, Jenna," Cody said. "You heard her. Go back and see her at the shop next time you're out shopping or come to see me for an appointment. Now back to your question, Maggie. Unfortunately, these wonderful cupcakes still contain carbs and should still be considered occasional treats. Remember, when you are diabetic, your body gets overwhelmed when you eat too many carbohydrates. The good news is that Jenna's low-carb cupcakes are filling and satisfying, and an occasional treat every couple of days won't hurt if you eat your optimal diet most of the time."

After another thirty minutes of answering questions, Cody and Kristin closed out the event, and the crowd slowly dissipated.

A few lingering guests who were waiting to talk to Cody stopped at her table and polished off the last of her samples. Most of them were thrilled they could finally buy tasty alternatives and still eat healthy. The only exception was Clarissa's friend, Marigold, who grimaced in disgust when she tried the lemon cheesecake sample. But then, Marigold never liked anything that wasn't a designer-brand or fancy enough to be labeled as a luxury item.

Jenna watched as poor Cody tried to make his way toward her, but the ladies wouldn't let him go.

Instead, she smiled and cleared her display table. Not a crumb of cupcake remained, which made cleanup a breeze. She stored her display trays and salvageable decor in the container she had stowed under the table and tossed the disposable tablecloth. By the time she had put on the lid, Kristin and her husband came by to see her.

"Jenna, you've done a wonderful job with your cupcakes. They are absolutely delicious. Do you have any of your business cards left? I want to hand them out to my clients."

"Oh, thank you so much. And yes, I do have a couple left." Jenna rummaged through her purse and gave her the small rubber-banded stack that had remained on the table. "I can send you more if you want."

"That's okay," Kristin said. "I'll be in town at least once a week helping Cody with his group meetings. If you ask me, he has some great ideas for his practice and the community, and I can't wait to see how they turn out."

"Well, you're welcome to come by the shop anytime," Jenna said. "Also, since you're a nutritionist, if you have any ideas about expanding the Doctor-Approved line, I would like to get your feedback."

"Deal," she said and reached out her hand.

"It was good to meet you," Jenna said, keeping her prior poor judgement to herself.

Kristin and Steve said goodbye to Cody on the way out, and his last guest left as well. They were finally alone.

Cody tucked his hands in his pocket and smiled as he walked toward her.

"Great turnout," Jenna said. "I think you won some of our locals over."

"It was much better than I had expected," he said. Cody stood in front of her, his eyes never leaving hers. "The only person I need to win over now is you."

Jenna's heart fluttered wildly in her chest. "Oh no, it's not that easy," she said. "You need to try a little harder than that."

He smiled. "That's fair. I'm sorry, Jenna, for all the grief I caused you," he said. "Can you forgive me?"

Jenna held her index finger against her chin. "Try harder."

Cody raked his hands through his hair. "You are a tough cookie, Miss Jenna," he said, and his facial expression turned somber. "To be honest, I appreciate how many chances you've given me," he began, "even though I didn't deserve them. Whatever it takes to regain your trust, I'll do. Because in these last few weeks, I've seen how hard you worked and how much the people of Magnolia Hill mean to you. I admire that in you. So, I ask, what can I do to make things well between us?"

Jenna rested her hands on her hips. "There is one—no, there are two things that would make me consider accepting your apology." She held up her index finger. "Promise me from now on to talk to me first when you get upset?"

"You've got it!" he said with a smile and a slight flush.

"Two," she continued. "A kiss," she said with a soft voice.

"Oh, Jenna," he whispered, his lips closing in on hers as he tucked that rogue strand of hair behind her ear.

Jenna closed her eyes. She felt his warm breath first on the tip of her nose, where he left a soft kiss. He then nudged her chin up toward him. Finally, his lips met hers, and he drew her into a tight embrace.

"I've been waiting for someone like you for a long time," he said as he held her against his chest.

"Me, too."

CHAPTER EIGHTEEN

"There ya go!" Cody said as he gave Jenna a boost up the wall obstacle in his ninja playground a month after the diabetes event. Her shoulder had healed faster than he had expected, and since this was the first pleasant Saturday afternoon in a couple of weeks, today was a perfect day for Jenna to come over and join him for a fun workout.

"Thanks for inviting me for a play date," she said, perched on top of the wall, her legs dangling in the air.

Cody couldn't wait for her to join him on the playground, but he wanted to make sure that her shoulder could handle it. The last thing he wanted was for her to re-injure herself. "Psst, don't tell anyone, but there's this woman in town wearing these frilly aprons and making amazing cupcakes. She had begged me for weeks to come and play on the ninja playground. But I always told her no." He winked at her.

Jenna laughed. "I heard about that woman. You know, rumor has it she's got a huge crush on you."

"Oh, does she?" he asked. "Did anyone tell her I'm already taken?" He then took a running start, gripped the top edge of the obstacle, pulled himself up, and stole a quick kiss before he jumped off on the other side.

"Well, Dr. Walker, I consider myself lucky that I made it in your exclusive circle of friends that are privileged enough to play on your fine playground."

Cody harrumphed. "Last I checked, friends don't kiss each other. I think we're past the friend-zone," he said with his arms stretched out toward her. "Come on down, I'll catch ya."

Jenna looked to the ground and then focused on him as she pushed herself off the top of the eight-foot wall and landed right in his arms.

Cody had to take a step back to balance himself, or they both would've gone down. He didn't want to let her go just yet, so he kept her tight in his embrace. "I think this workout will take a long time if we're going at this pace."

The corners of her mouth lifted into a mischievous smile as she pulled herself up toward him. "That's okay. We have all day to try out all the equipment. Besides, the next obstacle can wait," she whispered as she closed the distance between their lips, then kissed him.

"I could get used to this," he said when she pulled away.

Jenna suddenly turned and ran to the tire obstacle. "There's more of that after the next obstacle," she called out. "I race you!"

He laughed. "Not fair! You got a head start." Then he ran after her.

"You said nothing about rules."

He caught up with her just before she reached the eight

pairs of tires lined up ahead of them and reached for her waist. "Cheating will cost you another kiss," he said as she turned and leaned back in his arms, laughing. He pulled her closer to him again.

She wrestled herself out of his embrace. "Nope, you've got to earn it." She ran through the obstacle, stepping in each tire as she moved through, then exited the last tire with an elegant jump fit for an Olympian gymnast.

"Wow," he said. "She has mad skills, and grace too. I'm impressed." He wondered how many other surprises he'd discover as they got to know each other better.

"That's years of gymnastics as a kid until the money ran out."

"Did you compete?" he asked as he ran through the tires.

"Yep. I made regional champion two years in a row," she said, "but my parents ran into some hard times and couldn't afford the club fees and travel anymore."

"I'm sorry." But then also was glad that she didn't make it to an Olympic level. Training and injuries for this type of athlete could be hard on the body. He'd rather see her healthy with a strong quality of life, instead of her having to deal with chronic pain.

"It's all good," she said with a smile. "In the end, I still would've ended up opening my cupcake bakery."

"And I'm glad you did," he said, returning her smile. If it hadn't been for her, he'd still would've been stuck in his one-size-fits all, black-or-white philosophy. Because of her, he finally came to his senses and saw beyond his self-centered thinking. Jenna had opened his eyes and reminded him what small-town life was all about and how to connect with his patients. It took her stomping over to his practice and give him the worst tongue-lashing he had received since medical school before he understood that a doctor-patient relationship went both ways. Cody made a mental note never to make her upset again.

After they finished the last obstacle, he wrapped his arm around her shoulder, and they walked toward his back porch.

"That was a lot of fun," she said. "And I could get used to those reward kisses."

"So could I," he admitted.

They reached the porch and walked the couple of steps up onto the deck, then plopped onto the cushioned wicker loveseat.

Jenna put her feet onto the ottoman and leaned her head against his shoulder. "We should do this more often," she said.

"I agree," Cody said, then stroked her arm. The afternoon sun felt wonderful on his skin, almost as wonderful as Jenna cuddling up to him. His stomach gurgled. "Sorry about that," he said. "I should get the grill ready for our rib-eyes, but I just can't get myself to get up."

"Then stay here with me just a little while longer," she whispered, closing her eyes.

That's when he knew that he'd never would want to let her go.

EPILOGUE

Six months later, Jenna and Beth were both working overtime in the kitchen while Willow held down the fort in the shop. They barely could keep up with their baking, even though Clarissa's consigned pies and other baked goods helped.

"I think we're back at square one. We need more help," Jenna said.

"You're preaching to the choir," Beth said, topping the latest of their cupcake creations—the Willow Whirl, a yellow cake batter with pink dots and green and blue icing on top. "I think we need one more person helping in the kitchen and one more up front."

"We definitely can afford it now with Kristin's patients coming, too," Jenna said. "These Doctor-Approved cupcakes sell better than any others in the shop. Willow, can you hang a sign in the window for baker and sales clerk vacancies when you get a break between customers?"

"I will," she said. "But first, you got a visitor."

Jenna washed her hands, dried them, and smoothed

down her apron as she stepped into the shop. Behind a small crowd of customers, she saw Cody's head poking out.

He made his way to her, stepped behind the counter, and greeted her with a kiss. "I see you're busy as always," he said, "so I promise, I won't keep you long."

"How did your appointment with your cardiologist go this morning?" she asked.

"Perfect. I got a clean bill of health," he responded. "I also checked with my attorney, and we can now allow people to work out on the property legally after signing a waiver."

"That's wonderful news," she said.

The door chimes of the shop kept ringing as a crowd the size of half the town jammed into the small shop area of the bakery.

She noticed Maggie, Anna, Jason, Kevin, Sean, Twyla, and many more familiar faces. Suspicious, she glared at Cody. "What's going on? Are you up to something?"

Sean pushed his way through the crowd. "Make room! This is official law enforcement business," he said, holding a Cherry on Top box. "Here you go, Cody," he said and opened the lid for him.

With a cupcake towering with icing in hand, Cody bent down on one knee.

Almost faint, Jenna held her hands against her face. She glanced at Beth, who nodded.

"Jenna, I can't forget the evening of the tornado. That's when I got the first glimpse of who you really are. That evening opened my eyes, and ever since then, I wondered how I could ever win your trust back, if there was a way at all. Today, I want to deepen my commitment to you to make you the happiest woman in the world. I hope that by giving all of my heart and soul to you, you'd consider spending the rest of our lives together."

He held up the pink and gray cupcake, which was decorated with a sparkling diamond ring on a little stick. "Jenna, will you marry me?"

She couldn't hold back the tears. With a sniffle, she nodded. "Yes, Cody," she managed. "I will marry you."

He pulled the ring out of its holder and was about to put it on her finger when she pulled her hand back.

"Wait! Not so fast, Doc Walker," she said. "I have two more conditions I want you to make official with all these witnesses today."

"Name them," he said.

"One, a lifetime membership to your improved ninja playground."

A broad smile spread across his face. "You got it," he said. "Lifetime membership to OUR improved ninja playground is now approved."

"Two, I want an unlimited amount of your sweet kisses," she said with a smile.

"And then I can put the ring on you?" he asked. The corner of his lips turned up into a cheeky grin.

"Yes."

He turned to the people in the shop. "You all are my witnesses," he said, then turned his attention back to Jenna. "I, Cody Walker, promise you, Jenna Wilson, a lifetime membership to the ninja playground and unlimited kisses." He held his hand out for hers. "Now that it's official, will you marry me?"

Jenna nodded, then let him take her hand.

Cody slid the ring on her finger, then gently kissed her

to seal the deal.

The crowd in her shop hooted and cheered as he scooped her up into his arms.

"You should try the cupcake," Beth nudged her.

She removed the paper and took a bite. "Hm, what is it?"

"It's our new low-carb Whirlwind Strawberry Twister," Beth said. "It was inspired by your now fiancé."

Jenna held the cupcake up to him to take a bite. "You might have a future in cupcake decorating."

"I'd better stick to practicing medicine. To tell the truth, without Beth and Willow, my cupcake would've turned into another pile of crumbling cake held together by a paper liner and topped with a lopsided pile of icing. There was no way you'd say yes after seeing that disaster in a box," Cody said.

"I appreciate the effort," Jenna said, and followed it up with a quick peck on his lips. Then she admired the diamond ring that fit on her finger like a glove.

"Well, I hate to be a party-pooper," Sean said, "but I have to pack and get the truck ready for our father-son trip into the Smokey's tomorrow. Grady is already mad to leave Ashleigh for a week."

"He'll get over it, Sean," Anna said. "I have it worse, because I'll have grief-stricken teenage daughter at my house."

Sean shook Cody's hand. "Congratulations, my friend," he said, hugging Jenna. "And congrats to you, too. I know you've been waiting for this moment for a long time."

Jenna squeezed him. "I have." She looked up at him. "You know, Sean, I've got this vibe…"

"Nope, not me. And on that happy note, I'm heading out," Sean said and left.

"Well, excuse me, everyone," Cody announced, "but my fiancée and I will take the rest of the afternoon off."

"I'd love to, but I can't," Jenna said.

"Of course, you can," Willow said. "We've got you covered. You deserve a break."

"But…" Jenna protested.

Cody put his index finger on her lips. "No buts. I'm trying to make good on those unlimited kisses."

"Well, how can I resist, Cody Walker?"

~ This is the end of Book 2 ~
Read on with Book 3 - Fire Watch.

Hello dear reader,

Are you ready to find out who Sean falls in love with?
Then continue with Fire Watch, the next exciting story of the Southern Storms series. You won't be disappointed!!!

Again, if you haven't already, why not read my **free** novella, **FLOOD WATERS**? It's exclusive to my Stormies (newsletter subscribers) at **https://bit.ly/2VDYUOb**.

Again, thanks for reading Twist of Fate. Enjoy Fire Watch!

Hugs,
Lexie

ALSO BY LEXIE NICHOLAS

<u>Southern Storms Series</u>

All novels can be read as standalone stories.

Hurricane Beach Book #1

Fire Watch Book #3

Christmas Blizzard Book #4

Flood Waters

A free bonus novella exclusive to Lexie's mailing list subscribers. Never miss a new release. You can sign up here: https://bit.ly/2VDYUOb

Scan QR code with your phone camera for book details and where to purchase them.

ABOUT THE AUTHOR

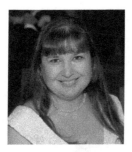

Lexie Nicholas is the author of sweet, small-town contemporary romances. She's a huge fan of Hallmark movies and recently also got hooked on K-Dramas.

Lexie lives with her husband, their dog, and their two cats smack-dab in the middle of the beautiful state of Alabama. Although it gets hot and muggy in the summer, the beach and inspiration are only a weekend-trip away.

Visit her at **https://lexienicholas.com.**

Want more? Lexie also writes sweet paranormal romances as Nickie Cochran—think Hallmark-style love stories with a fun ghostly twist.

Lexie loves to hear from her readers. You can find and follow her at these online places:

amazon.com/author/lexienicholas

facebook.com/LexieNicholasAuthor

instagram.com/lexienicholaswriter

bookbub.com/authors/lexie-nicholas

goodreads.com/Lexie_Nicholas